# HATHA YOGA
## FOR TOTAL HEALTH

# HATHA

# YOGA
# FOR TOTAL HEALTH

## HANDBOOK OF PRACTICAL PROGRAMS

by SUE LUBY

PRENTICE-HALL, INC., Englewood Cliffs, New Jersey 07632

*Library of Congress Cataloging in Publication Data*

LUBY, SUE (date).
  Hatha Yoga for total health.

  Includes bibliography and index.
  1. Yoga, Hatha.  I. Title.
RA781.7.L8      613.7      76-45473
ISBN 0-13-384107-3 case.
ISBN 0-13-384123-5 pbk.

**HATHA YOGA FOR TOTAL HEALTH**
**Handbook of Practical Programs**
by Sue Luby

Printed in the United States of America
10   9   8   7   6

PRENTICE-HALL INTERNATIONAL, INC., *London*
PRENTICE-HALL OF AUSTRALIA PTY. LIMITED, *Sydney*
PRENTICE-HALL OF CANADA, LTD., *Toronto*
PRENTICE-HALL OF INDIA PRIVATE LIMITED, *New Delhi*
PRENTICE-HALL OF JAPAN, INC., *Tokyo*
PRENTICE-HALL OF SOUTHEAST ASIA PTE. LTD., *Singapore*
WHITEHALL BOOKS LIMITED, *Wellington, New Zealand*

*I am dedicating this book to the students*
*whom I have had the pleasure of teaching for many years*
*and to those who have corresponded with me*
*after reading my first book,*
Yoga Is For You.

*Their appreciation and encouragement for my approach to Yoga*
*has been an inspiration for me*
*to write this extensive and comprehendible Hatha Yoga handbook.*

# CONTENTS

# PREFACE

Few people attain their full potential in the use and control of their bodies. Most let their bodies control them. In this book I teach *you* to control your body and not have *it* control you.

Through misuse and neglect people become flabby, out of shape, tense and lose flexibility and tone. For years man has studied how the body is put together and how it works. But only recently has serious consideration been given to how we feel about our bodies—how our body image and self-concept actually affect our behavior. I feel that a person's self-concept and body image very strongly influence his or her behavior. This individualized program helps a student learn how to reach his or her highest level of awareness, and work from that basic point, not pushing beyond the student's capabilities.

Self-image and social interaction depend to a large extent on self-perception and what can be done with it. By increasing your understanding and awareness of the correct ways of exercising, you improve in muscular strength, endurance, flexibility, agility, balance, and coordination. My aim in this book is to help you learn to control your mind and body in an intelligent manner so that your body will reflect a substantial gain in health and flexibility. This gain will allow you to project a positive, blooming self-concept. My approach to health encompasses the total person through Hatha Yoga, whose postures are designed to renew all parts of the body.

Our bodies are exhilarated by positive and negative currents. When these currents are in complete harmony, we enjoy perfect health. The name Hatha Yoga comes from the ancient language of the Orient. The positive current is designated by the letter "HA" which is equivalent in meaning to "SUN." The negative current is called "THA" meaning "MOON." The likeness can also be referred to left and right or backwards and forwards. The word YOGA means and is used as "joining," "union," and "yoke." Thus HATHA YOGA signifies the perfect knowledge of the two energies, the positive sun and negative moon energies, their joining in perfect harmony and complete equilibrium, and the ability to control their energies yoked within the control we have of our bodies.

Hatha Yoga, in contrast to other exercise programs, does not aim directly at muscular development, for it is a mistake to equate muscular development with a healthy body. In Hatha Yoga, health is defined as the state wherein all organs function perfectly under intelligent control of the mind. Each of us also has the capacity to use Yoga for improved health and appearance within an individual framework. It is therefore important to bear in mind that Hatha Yoga is noncompetitive. Do not compare your ability or progress with someone else's. You are uniquely and individually *you,* and you must not set impossible goals according to someone else's standards and accomplishments.

The Hatha Yoga approach is slow, smooth, and coordinated; movements flow to rhythmically controlled breathing. Although some of the postures may appear passive or relaxed, they are actually positive and dynamic. Slowly stretching muscles to full length and then holding them in absolute stillness causes blood to circulate evenly throughout the body. Hatha Yoga brings every muscle group into play. This allows the range of movement to be increased in all muscles, ligaments, tendons, and joints. Special emphasis is placed on increasing or renewing spinal flexibility by stretching. I often say to my students, "You are as young as your spine is supple." Therefore, a number of exercises have the express purpose of promoting the health, strength, and flexibility of the entire spine, from the cervical vertebrae in the neck to the lowest of the lumbar vertebraes. If you follow one of my regular Hatha Yoga programs, you will soon notice the "youth" returning to the spine and joints, where renewed flexibility can make all movement easier.

Hatha Yoga teaches deep, controlled breathing. This is as basic to the discipline as the emphasis on special body movements. Deep breathing is nature's tranquilizer and rejuvenator. Providing sufficient oxygen to the system wards off fatigue and sluggishness. Slow, deep respiration reduces strain on the heart and blood vessels. Lungs well exercised by proper breathing increase the body's ability to resist the common cold and other respiratory ailments.

I have designed this book to be used by beginning, intermediate, and advanced students. The flow of exercises is planned so that each student can progress to his or her own limit. Keep in mind that it is not how far you advance in a given posture that is important but that you perform each pose carefully and correctly to the best of your ability, gauging your progress solely against yourself—going only as far as you can while doing each exercise correctly. As you become familiar with each pose, you can write the tips you find most helpful in the space around the photos.

In my 13 years of teaching I have been fortunate in having an unusually rewarding relationship with my students. It is to all my students that I would like to acknowledge my thanks for their enthusiasm and support. The following are the students who were kind enough to pose for the pictures: Don Dion, Al Giglio, Ed Hasmer, and Bob Knox; Cyndy, Steve, and Ralph Luby; Don and Hilda Moss; and Mary Jo Murray and Terry Watson. I wish to express my deep and lasting appreciation to Hilda Moss, my loyal and wise advisor; Jane Vondell, for her dedicated assistance in editing; Fran McCormick, whose unique illustrations have greatly enhanced the reader's understanding; Ruth Williams, for her expertise as a Yoga teacher and photographer; Sandy Martinuk, for her patience and typing talents; and Dr. Kirt Josefek, for checking the anatomical details. Each person was indispensable.

Now let's begin to learn what I say to my classes: *You* control your body; do not let *it* control you.

# HATHA YOGA
## FOR TOTAL HEALTH

# 1 GETTING READY FOR HATHA YOGA

The best prescription for good health is proper breathing, daily exercise, proper rest, and the right diet. You can actually slow down the aging process by proper exercises; realize, therefore, that it is never too late to start looking and feeling younger, remembering what you don't use you lose.

There are hundreds of different Yoga postures. Some students will find that many of the postures require astonishing dexterity of the spine and limbs, for which long years of practice may be necessary.

People have the erroneous belief that these very difficult postures must be an intrinsic part of Yoga. They just cannot imagine their tired, tense, and stiff bodies executing some of the more difficult positions. They feel discouraged and naturally do not pursue the idea or the study of Yoga any further. But it is with these people in mind—those who desperately need a graduated Hatha Yoga program where every movement is completely natural and designed so they may start at their own personal level—that I have set the sequences in this book. Within each chapter the first posture or exercise is the warming-up and conditioning move, and one can move from there to accomplish correctly the more intricate postures that follow.

The most important fact to remember about this Hatha Yoga program is to execute each posture exactly as instructed. Study the technique, the photos and read the "tips" so you will visualize the exact placement of the body before you try any of the postures. When you just skim the instructions and do it in a sloppy manner you may be causing strain by involving the wrong group of muscles. When done correctly and with a systematic approach you will be incorporating a specific group of muscles, thus toning and strengthening them for better function, at the same time *removing* strain and tension from the body.

Do not allow yourself to get discouraged by attempting a posture chosen at random. I cannot say enough about the importance of the proper warm-ups;

for the beginner, the first and perhaps second posture of each chapter is important, for the experienced student, the All Inclusive Warm-Up Sun Salutation. You may think, "I only want to firm my tummy, so I'll skip the warm-ups." But please follow my advice. Never exercise unprepared or "cold" muscles; you might tear tissues or muscles. You will get better performance with minimum effort after you do the warm-ups; your body will feel warm and loose, ready for specific, concentrated postures.

Start by accomplishing the first of each group of postures. By starting from this beginning, you will be able to work from your own reference point, which is the point where you can feel your body move from within, without discomfort, and with a smooth flow of breath. You will find yourself limbering up from that reference point and feel an ease and freedom from within your body that will encourage you to challenge yourself just one step further. You must never strain to attain a position in which your body is uncomfortable. If you do so, you will actually retard your progress. The body is fully aware, challenging itself at all times yet holding itself in a wonderfully assured sense of balance and freedom. I often tell my students, "Don't strain! Reach up or stretch out only as far as you comfortably can, and then relax within the move. But before you come out of the pose, take one more breath and stretch just a little bit more. That's it. You just do what you can—and then challenge yourself a little bit further." Do the exercises *slowly* and with control, do not rush through even the warm ups. Yoga is as much to listen to your body as well as it is moving the body. Your body will tell you what condition it is in. You should differentiate between pain and aches. If you start off by doing too much you will only fatique the body. Ideally, a workout of ten to fifteen minutes a day is far better than one hour once a week. In the beginning you may feel a little achy when working muscles you haven't worked for some time. But with slow continual control and learning to relax *in* the posture the ache should pass. PAIN, though, is quite a different matter. It is telling us by signaling that something is wrong. When you feel this pain, stop immediately, lie down and relax applying some deep rhythmic breaths. Then check with your chiropractor, orthopedic or general physician. You may just have something out of alignment and with an adjustment can follow through with some corrective conditioning to build up the muscles in the weak areas.

An experienced Yoga student should move effortlessly, with simplicity and clarity of movement and breath. One is instinctive and fully aware of each movement executed. One knows the extent of movement in each part of the body—limbs, joints, muscles, and ligaments. With this awareness, one can move each separate part within its proper range, preventing jerkiness and thus create and produce a sequential flow of movement in the posture.

*Read the following points carefully before you begin your Hatha Yoga program.*

1. Although Yoga is considered to be nonstrenuous, it is always wise to check with your physician before embarking on any physical fitness program. If you have not had a recent checkup, you will be scheduled for an annual "physical," at which time you will be able to discuss this program's exercises with the doctor. The beginning exercises in each group are simple and undemanding. If you fall into the following categories, you should definitely get your doctor's permission before registering: abnormal blood pressure if it is abnormal for your age and condition, heart or circulation problems, and certain skull or eye conditions.

2. Good nutrition is a vital part of a good Hatha Yoga program. The Yogi is concerned, not with the amount of food he eats, but with the amount of life-force in that food. With three heavy, rich meals each day, one finds strength, vitality, and endurance decreased, and the mind functions less efficiently. Our organism is a precision instrument designed to function at its peak on small amounts of high-quality food. One grows more and more sensitive to the fact that light, high-quality foods can add to our life-force and help regenerate the body, whereas heavy, rich, or artificial food can sap our life-force.

The student should learn to eat only what is light,

agreeable, and fully nourishing; eat as many foods in their natural state as possible and avoid artificial stimulants, sugar, coffee, and alcohol. Read the labels on food to avoid artificial preservatives and sweeteners.

The Yoga student must make certain that his or her diet does not inhibit either the life-force already in the organism or the new life-force that will be gained through the Yoga postures.

3. Do not attempt to go on a starvation diet if you plan to lose weight. You should practice to eat small, good nutritious meals. Spend time practicing deep breathing. This stimulates and improves the metabolism, transforming deposits of fat into body fuel.

   Do not fast for more than two days without the supervision of an authority. I do not recommend fasting for everyone. Fasting is not starving. In fasting, you give up food for a certain amount of time as part of a regeneration program, during which time the digestive organs are allowed to rest and a cleansing process is initiated.

   For a partial fast, select a day when you can *rest* and *relax;* eat nothing that day. Simply drink pure water when you are thirsty. By fasting in this manner you are doing your body a great favor. The next day, always take small amounts of light, natural, and nourishing foods.

4. When our sleep is deep and restful, a powerful regeneration occurs, but most people pay little heed to how they can get the most from their sleep. They should sleep on a firm surface, head should be only slightly raised on a thin pillow to ease the neck into its natural curve. You should never sleep on your stomach but on your back or side with legs together (see my first book). Refrain from eating for two hours before resting. Follow the relaxation techniques at the end of this book for deep and restful sleep.

5. Smoking will inhibit your life, but do not force yourself to stop when beginning your Yoga program. Concentrate on practicing the breathing exercises and work on the postures until you can feel the nervous system grow calm and steady; then there will be no need for artificial tranquilizers of your nerves.

6. There is a misconception that you bend the body one way, then reverse, bending it the other way, and then bend back and forth. This will only cause stiffness. The correct way is to stretch the body, beginning with the first move within the chapter, and continue advancing that same stretching throughout the chapter. To rest or ease the spine, you may do any posture

in the Elongating Legs and Back chapter. Lie down and rest your body before going on to the next chapter, which will then stretch the body in a different manner. Basically all the postures are designed so that they are continually elongating the spine.

7. If you have a definite weak side and it is causing imbalance within your body, work up or out only as far as your weak side can perform. This way, you will be strengthening the weak side, instead of causing further imbalance by over-reinforcing the accomplishment of your good side. Soon both sides will be balanced, and your posture will improve.

8. Your daily check list:
   a) Wear loose comfortable clothing.
   b) Remove watch, rings, and any confining apparel.
   c) Have available your belt or tie, which measures a yard-and-a-half long.
   d) Have your beach towel ready and folded for a prop.
   e) Exercise on a semi-firm surface (ideally a foam mat, one-inch thick, and measuring 36" x 72"). Standing postures are to be done on the bare floor.
   f) Select a quiet, well-ventilated area away from the phone, with enough room to avoid having to move the furniture.
   g) Plan to devote 15 to 30 minutes to each day's practice. See back of book for schedule.
   h) The best time to practice is early in the morning before you are caught up in the day's activities.
   i) Before doing any exercises, wait at least two hours after a heavy meal, and one hour after a light snack.
   j) You inhale to get ready, and then exhale into the action of the posture. The breath and motion finish together.

9. Little Thoughts for the Day.
   a) The finality of a posture depends on the beginning.
   b) When the body is ready, you will be able to do the posture.
   c) Hatha Yoga is something living now—not in the past.
   d) Close your eyes to be self-aware, to experience, to feel—instead of using only the intellect.
   e) We have to feel—to see and understand.
   f) Like creating a vase in pottery, you cannot get to the top until the base is solid.
   g) A magnet stays far enough away to reach out, but not so far away as to lose control.
   h) As you give so shall you receive.
   i) A harmonious mind matches a rather slow and regular respiration.

A. Temporalis
B. Sternomastoid
C. Trapezius
D. Deltoid
E. Pronator Teres
F. Rectus Abdominis
G. Tensor Fasciae Latae
H. Adductor Longus
I. Gracilis
J. Vastus Lateralis
K. Extensor Digitorum Longus
L. Peroneus Longus
M. Frontalis
N. Platysma
O. Pectoralis Major
P. Biceps Brachi
Q. Brachiordialis
R. External Oblique
S. Extensor Carpi Radialis Longus
T. Pectineus
U. Sartorius
V. Rectus Femoris
W. Vastus Medialis
X. Tibialis Anterior
Y. Soleus
Z. Lateral Malleolus

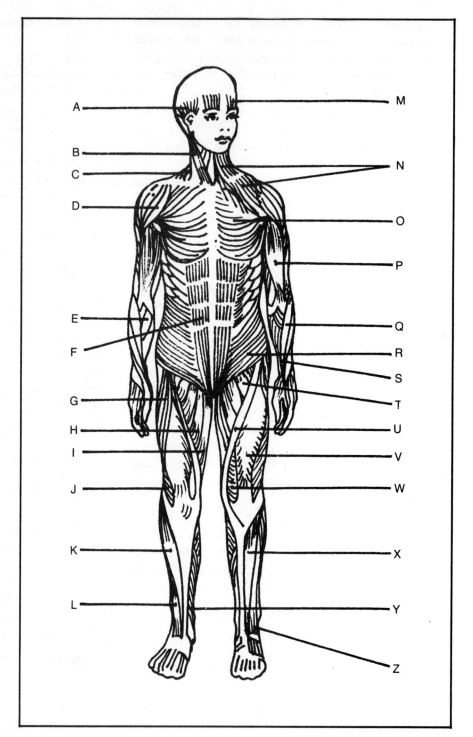

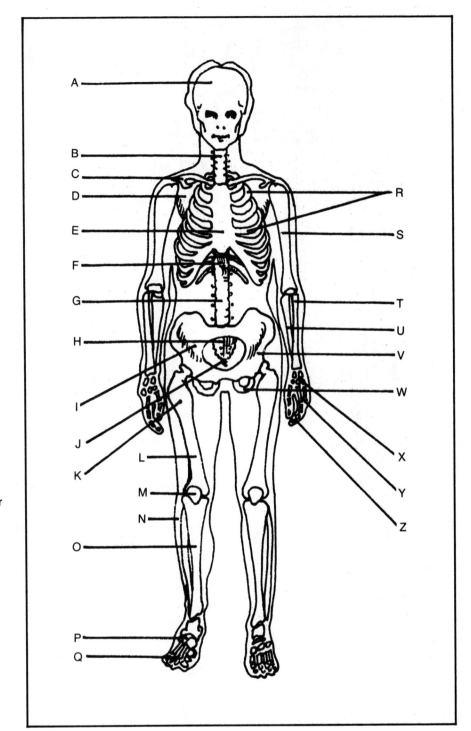

A. Skull
B. Cervical Vertebra
C. Clavicle
D. Scapula
E. Sternum
F. Thoracic Vertebra
G. Lumbar Vertebra
H. Sacrum
I. Ilium
J. Coccyx
K. Greater Trochanter
L. Femur
M. Patella
N. Fibula
O. Tibia
P. Tarsals
Q. Metatarsals
R. Ribs
S. Humerus
T. Radius
U. Ulna
V. Pelvis
W. Ischium
X. Carpals
Y. Metacarpals
Z. Phalanges

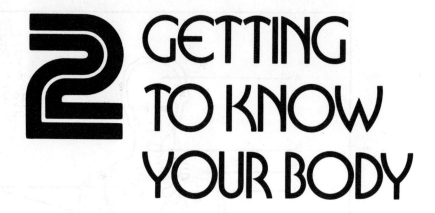

# 2 GETTING TO KNOW YOUR BODY

### *Getting to Know Your Body*

The human body is a marvelous creation that works for us under the best of conditions, and also under the worst, many of which we bring on ourselves by poor habits. The basic component is the skeleton, which consists of about 260 bones. More than 600 muscles are attached to the framework of the skeleton, and it is these muscles which hold us upright or move us through the almost infinite number of postures we assume in the course of a lifetime.

In Hatha Yoga, we are concerned with the bones and muscles because proper alignment of the body (a goal in itself) is necessary for proper execution of the postures. Correct alignment and breathing are the fundamentals of my teaching, and I will start by showing you how to align your body properly.

No doubt you have had experiences that are similar to mine with regard to body alignment, or as we call it "good" posture. Many times you were told or ordered by parents, gym teachers, or your drill sergeant, "Stand up straight! Suck in your stomach! Throw the shoulders back! Sit up straight!" Probably as many times as I was, and with the same results—an attempt at perfection that left you uncomfortable in much of your body. Most likely you were tense in your lower back, which you arched to support the upper body in this unnatural position. In my own personal search for this elusive ideal—perfectly balanced posture—I discovered that the place to begin to align the body is not from the top but from the feet.

Stand up and look at your own bare feet. Do you grip your toes? Is the weight all in the heels? Do your feet roll in and out? Do you feel any pressure in the small of the back?

There is a definite technique for the proper placement of the feet to support the body correctly.

6

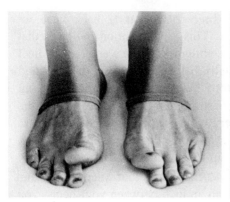
FIG. 2-1a

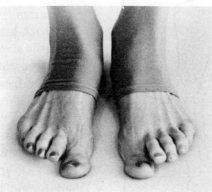
FIG. 2-1b

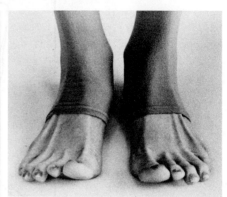
FIG. 2-1c

Stand straight, look at your feet and raise both your big toes, keeping your little toes on the floor, as in *FIG. 2-1a.* Hold for the count of 5.

Lower the big toes and raise the little toes, as in *FIG. 2-1b.* Hold for the count of 5.

Now raise all of your toes, while pressing the balls of your feet onto the floor, as in *FIG. 2-1c.* Hold.

The *weight should be evenly distributed between the heels and balls of your feet.* Relax the toes.

Now that your feet are based correctly, look at your knees. Are they sway-backed (hyperextended), knock-kneed, bowed, or crosseyed (tibial torsion)? I find that by noticing the position of my students' knees, I can almost "read" the areas where each body is out of alignment—so clearly do the knees reflect stresses and strains that may originate in faraway bones and muscles.

If the pelvis is off balance, with one hip higher than the other, it will show in the knees. A shoulder held habitually out of line may yield an out-of-line knee. Some of the stresses borne by the knee are the results of actual skeletal deformities, but most stresses have their origin in the many years of improper use of muscles and poor habits of motion or alignment.

The knees are the second "building block" in our series of alignment points. By positioning the knees in line with the feet, according to the instructions that follow, you will be able, perhaps for the first time, to feel what good posture should be. By working at it, you can eventually maintain good balance. Whereas correct alignment of the knees will not undo deformities of the bones or muscles, it will help to minimize certain defects by allowing other parts of the body to come into better balance.

There are four types of legs that require special care. When checking your leg alignment, you should not be misled by muscle contour but should visualize the bony skeleton underneath.

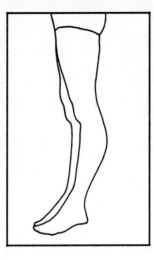

**Diagram 1**

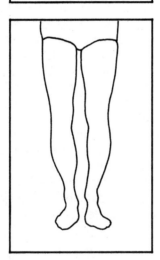

**Diagram 2**

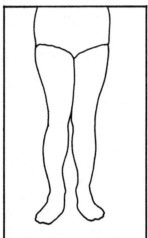

**Diagram 3**

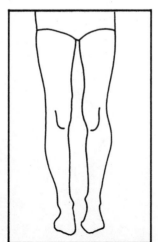

**Diagram 4**

1. *Hyperextended knee* **(DIAGRAM 1)**, back knee, or sway-back knee. This knee position indicates that the person stands with most of the weight on the heel rather than equally balanced between the heel and the ball of the foot. When my directions throughout the book indicate straightening the leg by raising the kneecap, be very careful not to lock the leg back. Instead, bring it forward to a straight position. Then raise kneecaps up toward the thigh.

2. *Knock-knee* **(DIAGRAM 2).** If your knees touch and there is more than an inch between your heels, you are knock-kneed. This can be more marked on one side than the other, causing an imbalance of the pelvis and a shortening of one leg. Whether or not there is a large amount of fat between the legs, a knock-knee condition is usually accompanied by over-rolling feet. Pay close attention to instructions on raising kneecaps and elongating the body. This will aid greatly in your postural alignment.

3. *Bowlegs* **(DIAGRAM 3)** are often the result of postural habits formed in early life. Causes include a) being encouraged to walk before the individual was ready and b) poorly fitted ice skates that caused one to skate on the ankles rather than directly on the blade. To check for bowlegs, stand with feet parallel and touching, weight forward, and knees comfortable. The amount of space between the knees determines the degree of bowlegs.

   To help overcome bowlegs, place feet together. Raise the kneecaps, tighten buttocks and tip the pelvis; this will bring ankles and knees together, Work also on exercises that stretch the hamstrings and keep paying particular attention to raising kneecaps.

4. *Crosseyed Knees* **(DIAGRAM 4).** If you stand with feet parallel, slightly apart, and find that your patellae (kneecaps) roll inward, you have crosseyed knees, a misalignment, but not one to be dismissed lightly. The slight correction of this imperfection can make a great deal of difference in balance for many postures. This is my area—my own crosseyed knees —where I have to work diligently.

   To help correct tibial torsion, stand tall, with feet together. Raise kneecaps, tighten buttocks, tip pelvis, and rotate thighs outward. When you attain proper alignment, relax the buttocks, but do not lose the lift and rotation of the leg.

   To feel the outward rotation of the thigh, do the following exercise. Lie face down, head resting on folded arms. Keep toes together and heels apart. Raise kneecaps. Slowly contract the buttocks as you deliberately bring the heels together. Hold and feel that rotation. Repeat until you feel that you can maintain the rotation while standing.

No matter what your "knee" category, follow through here, for even those with perfect bodies have to raise kneecaps. You will probably feel discomfort from the new placement because you have probably been out of line for a long period. As you practice the correctional exercises, your posture will improve and become more comfortable and balanced.

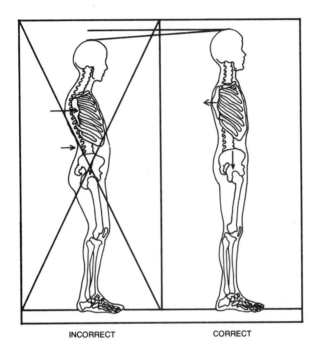

INCORRECT          CORRECT

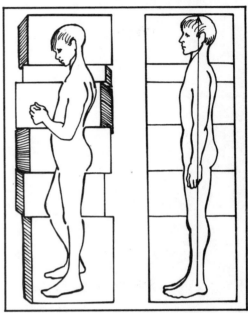

The first building block is the feet, the second is the knees, and the third is the pelvis. To continue aligning the body, tighten your buttocks to direct the pelvis into a balanced position, which is neither completely relaxed nor extremely tilted. If your feet and knees are positioned properly, this should not be difficult but should feel good.

Notice how much there is to the foundation of good posture. Only now are we ready to begin work on the upper body.

Lengthen at the waist, elevate the rib cage, and extend the sternum (chest bone). DO NOT THRUST THE CHEST OUT (forward). Do not shrug up but move the shoulders in the backward and downward movement toward the middle of the back (slight shoulder blade squeeze). Let the arms remain relaxed in this position. To complete the alignment, keep the back of the neck lengthened and held straight. To attain this, try to touch an imaginary hand 1 inch above the crown with your head. The weight of your entire body column should be equally distributed between the heels and balls of the feet.

With continued effort from this stable foundation, the spine can be lengthened not with muscular effort but by sensing. "Think tall" becomes reality. Learn to live 24 hours a day with a straight, aligned spine. Because of all of the anatomical irregularities, there are lapses into bad habits. It is very important that the student as well as the teacher consider and be aware of overall physical structures. If more caution and anatomical analyses were encouraged, the student would understand his own problem and could work from that level, instead of forcing his body into positions that are unnatural for him.

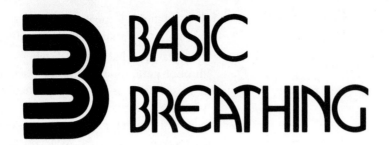

# 3 BASIC BREATHING

Deep, rhythmic breathing is the first lesson in Yoga and basic to all its teaching. This method of breathing literally feeds the body's tissues, organs, and glands with oxygen; removes much of body waste; and maintains good health, resistance to disease, and glandular balance. Deep breathing has a beneficial influence on the mind and emotions, relaxing the mind, clearing the memory, and promoting mental stability. In addition to these physiological and psychological benefits, breath control helps one gain a certain degree of mastery over the mind and body, for with each deep breath the individual incorporates a burst of energy, which expands self-expression and confidence as well as lungs.

Oxygen enters the body through the nose, where it is filtered, moistened, and warmed to avoid shocking the system. For this reason Yoga inhalation is performed with the mouth closed. The conditioned air continues its journey (to the lungs) through the passages shown in *DIAGRAM 1,* leaving finally from the last of a series of subdivisions of the airway, the microscopically tiny alveoli of the lung. These air cells, wrapped in plasma, are surrounded in a sac of plasma by blood vessels, nerves, and lymphatics, and it is here that the oxygen passes through from the lungs into the capillary walls and eventually to the arteries, which carry life-giving blood to the tissues. The waste (carbon dioxide) is carried from the blood in the veins, is exchanged through the capillaries into the alveoli, and is exhaled as the breath reverses the paths it took when it entered the nose.

The lungs, situated on either side of the thorax, are surrounded by the rib cage and bounded beneath by the diaphragm. Breathing is accomplished by the motions of the diaphragm and ribs. When exhaling, the diaphragm rises,

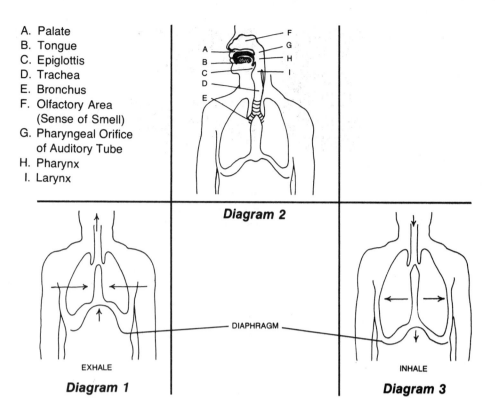

A. Palate
B. Tongue
C. Epiglottis
D. Trachea
E. Bronchus
F. Olfactory Area
   (Sense of Smell)
G. Pharyngeal Orifice
   of Auditory Tube
H. Pharynx
I. Larynx

**Diagram 2**

EXHALE

**Diagram 1**

DIAPHRAGM

INHALE

**Diagram 3**

pushing out the stale air up from the bottom of the lungs, as in **DIAGRAM 2.** When inhaling, the diaphragm lowers creating a vacuum deep into the lower lungs. The lungs fill first from the bottom with fresh air, working upwards expanding the ribs, and now up into the chest as in **DIAGRAM 3.** So remember, your nose and throat are just passage ways; keep them relaxed and open.

Westerners stress indrawing of the breath. Yoga, on the other hand, maintains that all good respiration begins first with a slow and complete exhalation then a complete full filled inhalation.

In my teaching I spend a great deal of time with each beginner, to see that he or she is breathing correctly. I feel this is the most important part of the whole Yoga program, but few teachers spend the time necessary to teach the student how to breath properly, much less to check on breathing progress.

Yoga recognizes three separate forms of breathing, each involving distinct segments of the respiratory apparatus, starting from the bottom up. Combinations of these breathing forms constitute the various Yoga breathing exercises.

*Diaphragmatic (or Abdominal) Breathing.* The air upon inhalation is drawn in, as the dome-shaped diaphragm muscle descends, pressing down on the abdomen and making it protrude slightly. The shoulders and chest do not rise. The exhalation is done slowly and evenly, drawing in the abdomen.

*Intercostal (Rib Cage) Breathing.* As its name implies, this is the action of expanding the thorax, and results from the inflation of the lungs when air is drawn into them. To perform Rib Cage Breathing properly, empty the lungs completely and keep the abdominal muscles contracted, so that it will be impossible to expand the abdomen with breath. Expanding the ribs outward as air is drawn in, thus filling the lungs. It is a breathing fault to experience ribs

*11*

expanding low in front; observe carefully, therefore, the sideways expansion. After a full inhalation the air is slowly and completely exhaled.

*Clavicular (Chest) Breathing.* As the air is drawn in, with only the upper part of the lungs receiving any fresh air, there is a characteristic breathing fault of many women who first raise their collar bone and shoulders, confining the lung area. But a Yoga student works at relaxing the shoulders and at the final stage of inhalation, concentrates on the clavicula and on extending the sternum.

*Complete Breathing.* This incorporates all three Yoga breathing methods, integrating them into one single, full, and rhythmic movement. Once the student has experienced all three stages of this method, the technique is refined by smoothing it out. Exhale before you begin to inhale. Now relax the abdomen as there is a slight wave of motion from the lowering of the diaphragm, which draws the air to the bottom of the lungs. The wave of motion moves upward as the ribs respond by moving toward the back and out sideways, feeling the lungs expand from within the ribs. When the inhalation seems complete and the lungs filled, a slight extension of the sternum occurs (note—still more intake of air). This upward extension of the sternum is very important, for in the many postures that require elongation of the torso, the leading point of the move is (from) the extended sternum. Exhalation now follows by contracting the abdomen, which raises the diaphragm upward, pushing out the air. To aid in emptying the lungs, also contract the ribs, eliminating any remaining stale air.

It is important to make this complete breath flow in a slow, smooth, fluid, continuous rhythm. I have seen too many students who have taken just a few Yoga lessons or have read the first part of a book and have never gotten past the first stage of the Complete Breath, and as a result they always breathe with a protruded abdomen. They not only find it difficult to exercise with a bulging tummy but also find themselves exhausted because they are using only one-third of their breathing capacity.

Breathing exercises are usually done in a room or studio that is clean and ventilated but free of direct drafts. For an optimum experience go outside each morning and take some complete breaths. For the first few days do not take more than 2 Yoga Complete Breaths a day. Gradually increase the number up to 60 full breaths a day. This should be a slow process, and you should take quite some time before the full quota of 60 a day is attempted. Be content at first to take just a few Complete Breaths at a time, for an overeager approach to deep breathing in a body unaccustomed to ingesting large amounts of energy can cause lightheadedness, dizziness, or other symptoms of hyperventilation. Please observe this word of caution, and work gradually and comfortably to the full daily quota of Complete Breaths.

The breathing that one would do throughout a whole day would not be as concentrated as one Complete Breath, but would still allow the lungs to fill using a deep natural rhythmic action involving the entire torso.

In executing the breath while exercising, the rate of breathing should adjust to the effort. The larger the effort, the deeper the inhalation.

When I teach, I call this complete method of breathing Rib Cage Breathing because I want to encourage students to expand their ribs to their fullest, to make them move their ribs at the side and back and reeducate them to avoid just "belly" and "chest" breathing. We want to work to fill our complete lungs.

Just as an accordion cannot be forced to fill or empty abruptly but must be drawn apart or squeezed gradually to accommodate air, so do the lungs and ribs react during rib cage breathing. If the student will keep this analogy in mind, Rib Cage Breathing will progress in a smooth and relaxed manner. Again, visualize the accordion and how the musician begins his song with the instrument empty of air, starting with an empty instrument, which is then filled by an intake of air. Similarly, normal respiration—and most especially Yoga breathing—begins with a slow, calm *exhalation,* to completely empty (receptacles of) the lungs from stale air before filling them afresh with the energy needed to perform. Always exhale calmly but deliberately before beginning a new round of breathing.

We take the act of breathing for granted. Learning how to breathe properly is basic to the performance of sports, gymnastics, dancing, and all exercise programs, but unfortunately proper breathing is often neglected in physical training curricula. The nonathlete also receives benefits from proper breathing. The educated inhalation nourishes starved tissues, and helps to normalize weight in those who are overweight or underweight; and the proper exhalation aids the body in ridding itself of wastes that have accumulated as fat or toxins.

Once you learn the correct way of breathing, begin the day with some deep, slow breaths while lying in bed—before you get up. Take advantage of every chance to be outdoors. During the day, at work or elsewhere, remember to take time for some deep Rib Cage Breaths. When you practice your "asanas" (postures), remember to synchronize the timing of your deep breaths in rhythm with the motion of your body. At the end of the evening take a few moments for a short session of breathing in bed. You will probably fall right to sleep.

Taking time to assimilate short but frequent sessions during the day will become a habit, and you will soon find yourself breathing the correct way most of the time. Complete Breathing will produce a healthier and cleaner body, a clearer and calmer mind, and a heightened spirit.

## TECHNIQUE

1. Sit with a straight spine with your *mouth closed throughout.*

2. Concentrate on the back wall of your throat.

3. Arrange the inside of your mouth and throat so that the tip of the tongue presses lightly against the back of the upper front teeth and the throat is open as if you were stifling a yawn.

4. Remember to keep the nose and throat open and relaxed. If it is difficult for you to breathe without a sniffing sensation in the nose, envision the air also entering through the ears, concentrating deep into the throat or hum in and out to get the proper sensation in the throat *not* the nose.

5. To exhale, contract the abdomen, which assists in raising the diaphragm upward, pushing out the stale air from the bottom up. Now, contract the ribs to further deflate the lungs. Relax the throat and nose, the air just escapes from the motion of the diaphragm and ribs.

6. To inhale, relax the abdomen and as if there were a suction pump at the base of your lungs (this being the diaphragm lowering and creating a vacuum), drawing the air deep into the bottom of the lungs. Concentrate on "aiming" at the center back of the lowest ribs. As the lungs inflate the ribs expand toward the back and out to the sides. When you feel the lungs can not expand any further sideways, extend your sternum and continue to fill the lungs to the top. The nose and throat are still relaxed. Remember, they are just passage ways, the inhalation and exhalation is the work of the diaphragm and ribs.

7. Think again of an accordion. (You can not force it open or shut, so do not rush your breathing.) In the beginning it should be done deliberately and smoothly going through each stage, letting the suction sound be clearly heard.

8. Ready! Place your hands on the side of your ribs, with thumb towards the back, *mouth closed,* back of the throat open. EXHALE to the count of 8, drawing in the abdomen and as the ribs contract apply pressure with the palm of your hand, as in *FIG. 3-1a* and *3-1b,* to completely let out all carbon dioxide.

9. Hold to the count of 2. It should be a natural pause. Do not be tense.

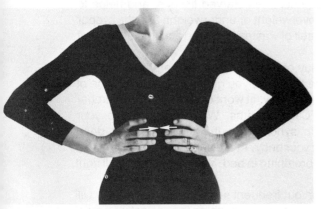

**FIG. 3-1a**

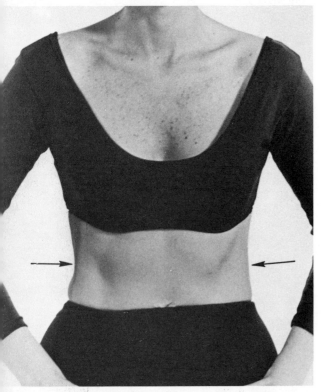

**FIG. 3-1b**

10. INHALE to the count of 4, relaxing the abdomen as you draw in the fresh air, letting the ribs expand outward; not up in front, but out from the sides and back, as in **FIGS. 3-1c** and **3-1d.** To complete the inhalation, extend the sternum. This will completely fill the lungs.

11. Repeat this, working to have both the inhalation and exhalation flow in a slow, smooth, fluid rhythm. If the suggested rhythm of 8 (exhale; hold to count of 2; inhale to count of 4) is not comfortable for you, work slowly at your own rate and gradually build up to it.

### TIPS

1. Continue this way until the ribs respond in rhythm with the inhalation and exhalation. Then relax arms and concentrate on breathing internally.

2. As you improve, there will be a need to increase gradually the duration of your inhalation, hold, and exhalation to a timing that is natural for you.

3. Remember to blend these 3 stages of breathing so they will flow. No staccatos!

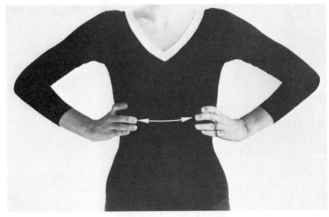

**FIG. 3-1c**

4. Really work to relax yourself and the throat and just *let* the air come in. If you rush it or try to force your body, you constrict the capacity. (Remember the accordion.)

5. Some beginners cannot relax their torsos while sitting up, and so for them breathing is begun lying down.

6. To experience the proper feeling of filled lungs with the ribs properly expanded sideways (from the back), make a tight roll with a hand towel. Lie down with this roll placed the long way between the shoulder blades. This will prop the back into the position where the sternum is extended and the shoulders rotated backwards and will allow the rib cage to expand properly with inhalation. Do Complete Breaths with this aid until you can reproduce the correct placement when the torso is upright.

7. This is the breathing that you will do while doing your postures.

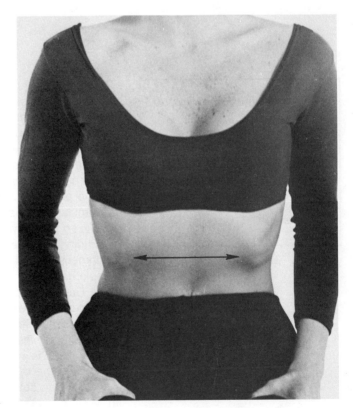

**FIG. 3-1d**

# 4 THE ABDOMEN AND PELVIS

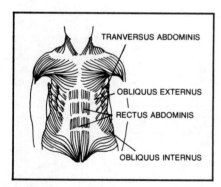

TRANVERSUS ABDOMINIS

OBLIQUUS EXTERNUS

RECTUS ABDOMINIS

OBLIQUUS INTERNUS

The abdominal muscle group is one of the most important groups involved in the movement of the spine. In exercising the abdominal musculature one should remember that the pelvis must be stabilized to obtain the maximum results in developing the abdominal muscles.

Before they were aware of the Yoga approach to exercises, many people who seek bodily self-improvement went through routines that gave them a series of movements to tone the abdominal muscles, but they never learned how to place the lower back properly to stabilize the pelvis. Repetition of abdominal exercises (sit-ups, leg raises, etc.) without a tipped, tilted, *stabilized* pelvis will result in the reinforcement of low back weakness and a protruding abdomen. Unfortunately, many exercised conscientiously to flatten abdomens made flabby by pregnancy, weight change, or neglect, and these people have only added to their problem.

The stable pelvis is tipped or tilted and will not flex past the designated point to obtain the maximum results in developing abdominal muscles. Among the major muscles that control this area and are to be exercised are these: *Rectus Abdominis Muscles* assist in flattening the lumbar curve and pull down on the ribs. It is important to observe that these muscles control the tilt of the pelvis and the curvature of the lower spine. *Obliquus Externus Abdominis Muscles* are a set of muscles that work on each side of the abdomen. They aid in twisting the trunk when they are working independently of each other. In working together they aid the rectus abdominis muscle in its action (right side of muscle twists to left). *Transversus Abdominis Muscle* forces expiration by pulling the abdominal wall inward. *Obliquus Internus Abdominis Muscles* run diagonally in the opposite direction to the obliquus externus.

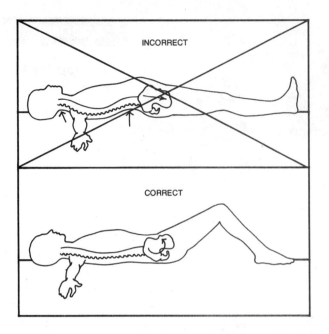

In tipping, the small of the back rests as flat on the floor as possible. The coccyx (tail bone) is on the floor, trying to curl upward toward the pubic bone, which should be drawn toward the sternum. The proper position would be the "tuck-under" used in postural alignment when one is standing.

The pivotal point for tilting the pelvis is at the hip bone. I have my students visualize this bone as a gear or crank, which is to be rotated toward the upper body.

In addition to the rotation at the "gear" of the hip, which gives the feeling that the coccyx and pubic bones are somewhat up and the sacroiliac down, the abdomen itself must be relaxed and pulled in; this is a seeming contradiction. To accomplish this, lie on the back with knees bent just hip-distance apart. Inhale, bring the arms down so the hands push downward against the hip bones. Exhale as you rotate the shoulders back and push down against the hip bones, rotating your hip "gear" to tip the pelvis to its utmost. At the end of the exhalation, allow the diaphragm to go up under the ribs (tummy-in) by using a mock inhalation before taking a real inhalation. This will pull the tummy and viscera up under the rib and the navel toward the spine. Assume this position whenever you prepare to do any exercise that starts in a supine position (unless otherwise directed), especially for those involving abdominals or lower back. This pelvic tipping is used in almost all postures, and the proper stabilization of this area is vital to the success or failure of a tummy-firming program.

Leg raises are a basic lower back/abdominal muscle therapy. Go back again to the "gear" at the hip bone and visualize the leg itself as a crane that you are trying to raise with a chain (the muscles). Many leg raises done in good faith neglect to stabilize the pelvis by rotating the "gear" to form a pivot in which the force of the muscles (chains) is focused to raise the leg (crane). The work of raising the legs comes not from the leg but from the tipped, rotated, stabilized pelvis on which the abdominal muscles then rest in perfect position, to be exercised without popping out or pulling up on the lower back.

The belt is used in leg raises to maintain the elongation and stretch of the leg muscles from the extended heel to the thigh. In this fashion, the muscles are not slack, and the strain on the abdomen is lessened.

Persons who suffer from a bad back, protruding stomach, sway-back, weak leg muscles and shallow breathing should give attention to exercises that strengthen the abdominal area.

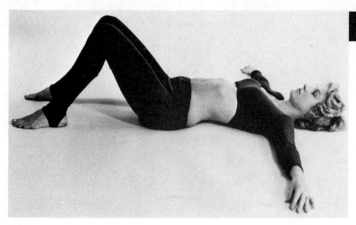

FIG. 4-1a

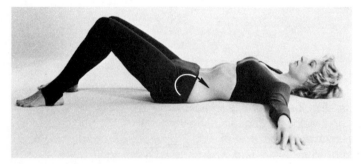

FIG. 4-1b

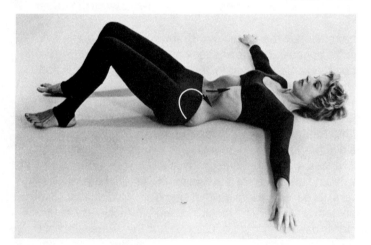

FIG. 4-1c

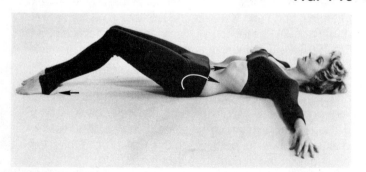

FIG. 4-1d

## Tipping Pelvis

### TECHNIQUE

1. Lie down on your back. Most everyone has some sort of arch, as in *FIG. 4-1a,* and if you continue to do the exercises without properly placing the back on the floor, you will not only weaken the tummy muscles but also strain your back. So with this understanding, let us really apply the steps that follow.

2. Bend your knees and tip your pelvis, rotating the tip of your spine toward the ceiling as you lower the small of the back to the floor (*FIG. 4-1b*). Exhale and pull your tummy in (*FIG. 4-1c*) without inhaling. Then you may resume normal breathing. But as you inhale, expand the ribs out to the side, not letting the tummy float down past the waist.

3. Keeping your pelvis tipped as you slowly lower your legs to the point just before your back wants to come up (*FIG. 4-1d*). Some of you may find that your feet are lower than in this picture or not as low.

4. At this point, reinforce keeping your back on the floor with a stronger tip, making sure your tummy remains in. This will all work smoothly if you keep an elongation within the spine.

5. Practice Steps 1 through 4 until they become an automatic procedure whenever you must tip your pelvis while lying down or standing.

## Abdominal Lift Warm-Up

### TECHNIQUE

1. Lie down on your mat with legs hip-distance apart. Bend your legs at the knee until your feet are flat on the floor (see *FIG. 4-2a*).

2. Complete two good rib-cage breaths. After the third inhalation, which leaves the sternum up and shoulders down, forcefully blow out *all* the air that is in your lungs without popping the tummy in and up, until your ribs are completely contracted *(FIG. 4-2b)*.

3. Draw your tongue back against the roof of the mouth, forming a "valve" to lock the air out. Do not inhale again until you have completed the whole exercise.

4. Tip your pelvis (as you pull the whole abdominal region back toward the spine) and lift it up toward the breastbone. To elongate, push away with your hands on your hips *(FIG. 4-2c)*. This will aid in further tipping your pelvis, bringing your spine completely flat to the floor.

5. Once you have accomplished the proper abdominal grip, feel the vacuum in your throat. Take advantage of this vacuum by tightening the buttocks slightly and attempt to pull the abdomen in and up a little further. Hold for the count of 5. Now you may relax the stomach and inhale *(FIG. 4-2d)*. Take 2 slow Rib Cage Breaths to normalize your breathing.

6. Repeat 2 more sets, but make sure you relax between each set.

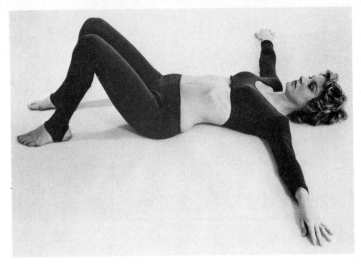

**FIG. 4-2a**

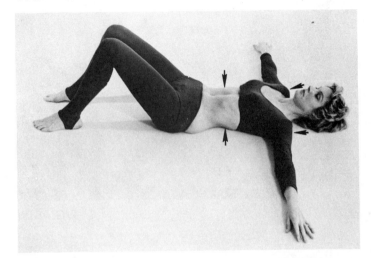

**FIG. 4-2b**

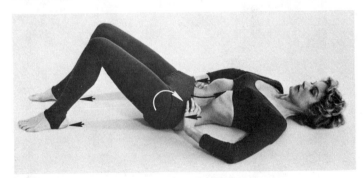

**FIG. 4-2c**

**FIG. 4-2d**

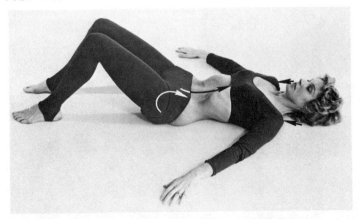

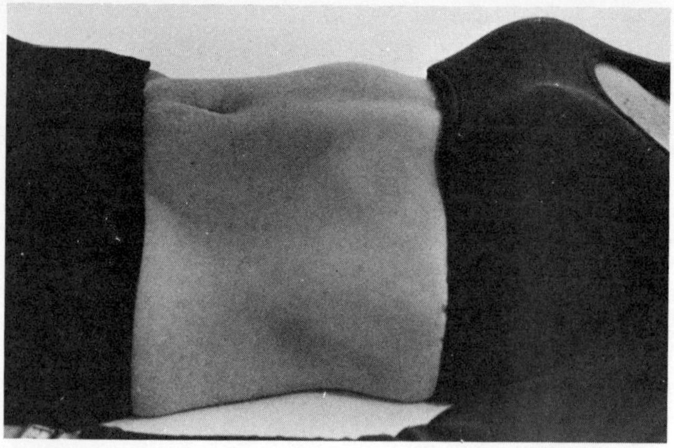

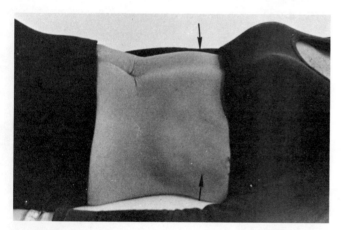

FIG. 4-3a

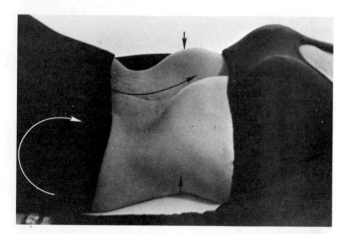

FIG. 4-3b

### TECHNIQUE

1. You now have warmed up and know how to control your abdominal muscles. This Tummy-In procedure is what you will apply while doing your exercises.

2. Relax, as in *FIG. 4-3a,* with arms beside the body. Inhale, extending the sternum. Exhaling, contract the abdomen and ribs, rotating the shoulders down to the floor. Continue to exhale, tightening the buttocks. Keep the sternum up while the ribs are completely contracted *(FIG. 4-3b).*

3. *Do not inhale.* Tip pelvis, apply a *mock* inhalation, and lift the tummy up toward the breast bone *(FIG. 4-3c).* When this is accomplished, let your breath flow into a deep inhalation *(FIG. 4-3d).* This "Tummy-In" action should flow right into a smooth inhalation. There should not be a strong gasping for breath.

4. Be aware of your lungs filling up and the ribs expanding out to the sides. Note: pelvis is still tipped and tummy flat. Keep your shoulders relaxed throughout this whole posture.

5. Repeat until you can inhale and exhale smoothly while applying the Tummy-In action. This is a basic procedure throughout this book and must be followed to execute these postures correctly, with one exception (a posture where you are lying *on* your abdomen).

FIG. 4-3c
FIG. 4-3d

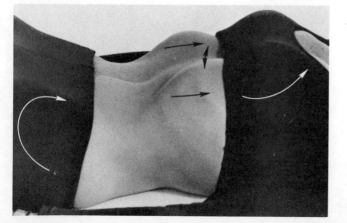

*TIPS*

1. Make sure that your feet are in the proper position, not too close to the buttocks.
2. For the Abdominal Lift Warm-Up, you must apply effort and force in completely blowing all the air out of your lungs. This is most important and will enable you to get the proper lift.
3. If you find yourself coughing, you must have inhaled slightly, so check this tendency the next time.
4. For the Tummy-In Warm-Up, do not contract the abdomen so much that you gag when you inhale. This procedure should flow smoothly into an inhalation and become natural.
5. A good rule to remember is to apply a "Tummy-In" action after each exhalation, thus creating that elongation one needs in each posture while inhaling.
6. In both variations, when exhaling and contracting the abdominal muscles and the rib cage, keep elongated and concentrate on keeping your tummy from popping up. It will become easier as your muscles strengthen and you acquire the discipline.

*BENEFITS*

Aids in elimination.
Firms and strengthens the abdominal muscles.
Tones the skin and abdominal organs.

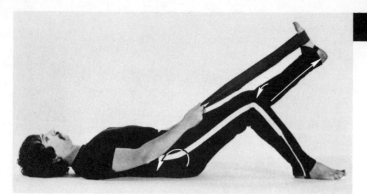

FIG. 4-4a

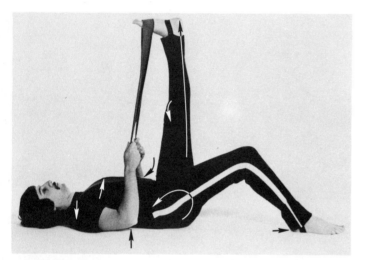

FIG. 4-4b

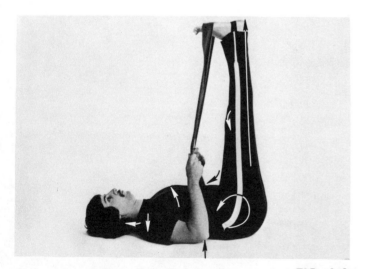

FIG. 4-4c

### Single Leg Raise

*TECHNIQUE*

1. Lie down, bend your knees. Bring the left knee to the chest as you place the belt around the ball of the left foot. Straighten the leg, raising the kneecap toward the thigh. Lower the leg so both knees will be level with each other *(FIG. 4-4a)*.

2. Inhale in this position, extending the heel. Exhale, contract the abdomen and ribs, tipping your pelvis, raise your leg so it will be straight up toward the ceiling *(FIG. 4-4b)*.

3. Without moving your body, push away, with your right heel sliding your coccyx back along the play in the skin until the play stops. (Think of the manner in which your skull and scalp move.)

4. This will further tip your pelvis. After having completely exhaled, apply the Tummy-In action, flowing into an inhalation. With a straight leg, extend the heel higher.

5. Adjust the hand grip so your elbows are beside the body and only about 1 inch off the floor (see *FIG. 4-4b*).

6. Apply the Tummy-In action, tipping your pelvis. Exhale, extending the whole left leg but not so much that the buttocks leave the floor. Feel the elongation from within the hip.

7. If you have mastered the above with your back flat, tummy in and no tension, you may remove the belt. Make sure you maintain good abdominal control, with it firm and not protruded. And keep the leg vertical and straight.

8. Inhale once again. Exhale, lower the left leg with extended heel. Just lower it to the point where both knees are level, then bend at the knee, placing the foot on the floor. Repeat with the right leg, and work each side 2 more times.

### Double Leg Raises

*TECHNIQUE*

1. Bend both knees to the chest. Place the belt around the balls of both feet.

2. Inhale. Exhale as you raise, and then straighten out the legs *(FIG. 4-4c)*. Adjust arms (Step 5).

3. Inhale, apply the Tummy-In technique as you extend the heels, keeping the kneecaps raised toward the thigh.

4. Exhaling, shrug your shoulders down and away from the ears, elongate the back of the neck so chin is not up in the air, while feeling the spine flat on the floor.

5. Take 3 rhythmic breaths in this position. Inhale while extending the heel and exhale while contracting the abdomen and ribs. Shrug your shoulders down. Do not let your tummy pop throughout this posture.

6. As you acquire good abdominal control, you will find you don't need the belt. So take it away *(FIG. 4-4d)*.

7. Inhale once again. Exhaling, extend the heel, maintaining the tipped pelvis; slowly lower the legs. Only lower them to the point where your lower back remains on the floor and your tummy can stay in.

8. Just before you feel you are about to lose control, bend at the knees, bringing the feet to the floor. Take a few breaths to relax, and you may repeat if you wish.

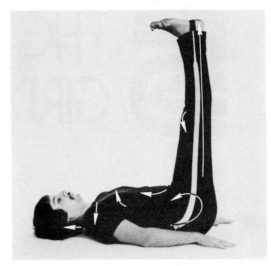

*FIG. 4-4d*

### TIPS

1. Make sure the belt is at the ball of the foot. Don't let it slip to the arch.

2. Be sure to shrug the shoulders down toward the floor and away from the ears on each exhalation. On each inhalation, after the Tummy-In approach, extend your sternum upward. This will aid in your breath capacity and rotation of the shoulders.

3. In the beginning do not attempt to raise or lower both legs from the floor. (This is not what I instructed in the previous steps.) This will only strain the lower back. Only when you can do the steps described above without a belt and can lower the legs to the floor, keeping the lower back flat and tummy in, are you ready to even try. If your tummy pops and your back comes up from the floor, you are not ready.

4. Concentrate on stretching the muscles up the back of the leg as you extend the heel. This will eliminate cramps in the front thigh.

5. Inhale and exhale to the count of 4 throughout this exercise, with the exception of the last exhalation, where you exhale to the count of 8 in coordination with lowering the leg.

### BENEFITS

Strengthens lower back.
Tones and firms abdominal organs.
Relaxes legs and helps vein and artery conditions.

# 5 THE SHOULDER GIRDLE

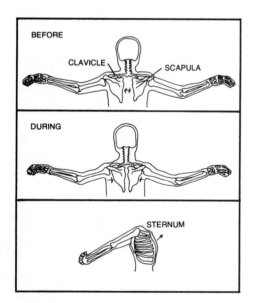

BEFORE

CLAVICLE    SCAPULA

DURING

STERNUM

Poor postural habits and faulty breathing are the usual reasons for the failure of thorax and shoulder girdle muscles to work properly. The value of breathing deeply is not so much for the effect on the lungs as for the mobilizing effect of the chest wall and even of the spine.

Students who study dance or conditioning for a sport concentrate to a greater degree on the building up of their legs and strength and often neglect the importance of developing a good chest and proper breathing habits.

The sagging, narrow chest makes the student tire easily and prone to injury in the thoracic spine. A brief sketch of the anatomy of this area will serve to illustrate the dependency and interaction of all of its parts.

The arms are attached to the body by means of the shoulder girdle, which is formed by the union of the clavicle (collar bone) with the scapula (shoulder blade). The clavicle connects with the sternum (breastbone).

The postural deviation most common to shoulder girdle is "round shoulders." This results from weakness in the muscles that hold the scapula against the upper posterior thoracic wall. People who are abnormally tense in this area tighten these muscles to an extreme, creating rigid shoulders, and thus affect the entire body alignment.

The skeletal diagram of the blade shows the scapula (shoulder blade) moving toward your spinal column and down, using muscles of the upper back—not the arms—and putting the sternum into correct position, which is diagonally forward and up.

By executing the following postures, you will be developing and strengthening the thorax and shoulder girdle. You will find movement freer, posture improved, and breathing more natural. You will also find yourself gaining flexibility in the spinal column, arms, and pelvic girdle.

Remember to take good complete Rib Cage Breaths while in the "hold" position. This will develop your breathing capacity.

## TECHNIQUE

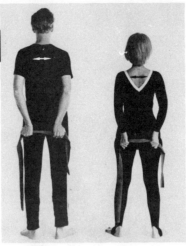

FIG. 5-1a

1. As in **FIG. 5-1a,** stand straight, feet slightly apart, clasping onto a belt with hands hip-distance apart. Note that the palms of the hands are toward the buttocks.

2. Inhale, extending sternum, then exhale as you shrug your shoulders down and back away from the ears. Relax your neck. Stretch downward with your belt as you rotate elbows inward, until they are straight, as in **FIG. 5-1b.**

3. Inhale, then elongate, extending the sternum. As you exhale, shrug the shoulders back further to feel a tighter squeeze down between the shoulder blades. You should never feel tension up in the neck.

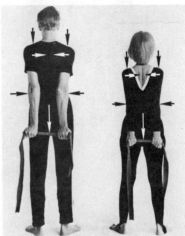

4. Keep this squeeze throughout this pose. Inhale, once again extending sternum, and this time, while exhaling, keep the squeeze as you raise your arm up, as in **FIG. 5-1c.** Do not sacrifice the tight shoulder squeeze, the elongation and the extended sternum by trying to go up too far.

5. When you find your spot, inhale and extend sternum; exhale as you shrug the shoulders back further. Slowly come down and do this for 3 more rounds.

FIG. 5-1b

## TIPS

1. If you find that you are arching your back, tip your pelvis. It is important to stand straight.

2. If you want more squeeze, slide your hands closer together on the belt.

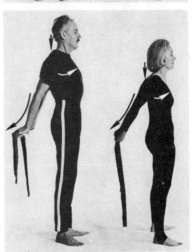

3. When you can do this with the hands touching on the belt, you are ready to do it without the belt. Clasp your hands behind you with palms open, then together, as in FIG. 5-1d. Start over from Step 1 and proceed.

FIG. 5-1c

## BENEFITS

The chest is expanded well and breathing becomes fuller.
Improves posture, correcting rounded shoulders.
Relaxes muscles of neck, shoulders, and upper back.

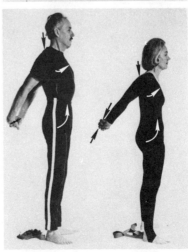

FIG. 5-1d

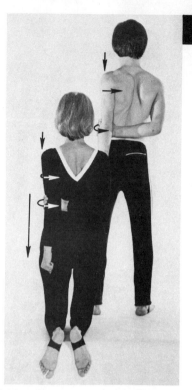

**FIG. 5-2a**

## TECHNIQUE

1. You can either stand or kneel, but you must keep a straight spine.

2. Make a fist with your left hand. Straighten the left arm. Shrug your left shoulder to the back and down, away from the ear.

3. Bend your right arm at the elbow. From behind, take hold just above the left elbow. Do not bend at the left elbow. Inhale as you stretch tall. Exhale as you shrug the left shoulder back and feel the left shoulder blade pulling in toward the center, as in *FIG. 5-2a.* Hold for the count of 5 and repeat for the opposite shoulder blade.

4. You are now warmed up for the Blade. Inhale as you outstretch your arms to the side at shoulder level. Do not let your shoulders come up toward the ears as in *FIG. 5-2b.* Keep them down. Exhaling, extend the

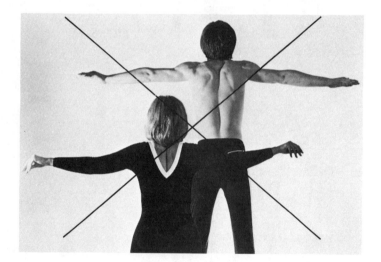

**FIG. 5-2b**

hands out to the side as far as possible, feeling them lengthen, as in *FIG. 5-2c.* Hold for the count of 5.

5. Now, without moving your arms back and with relaxed wrists and elbows, exhale as you draw your shoulder blades in together as though pressing a coin between them, as in *FIG. 5-2d.* Hold tightly for the count of 5. Do not tense the neck. Release and lower the arms slowly. You may repeat Steps 4 and 5 four times.

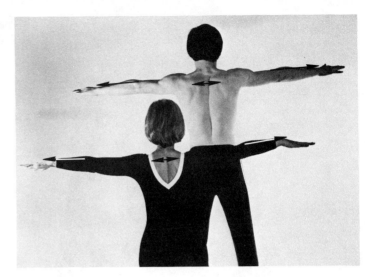

*FIG. 5-2c*

## TIPS

1. Do not shrug the shoulders up toward the ears.
2. Do not allow arms and shoulders to wobble up and down.
3. The extended arms must be completely straight, but when making a Blade Squeeze, the elbows bend only very slightly.
4. Shoulder blades pinch only toward one another and then back again. The arms do not move in and out.

## BENEFITS

Firms the upper back and pectoral muscles.
Reduces bursitis and arthritic pain.
Eases tension in the shoulders and upper back.

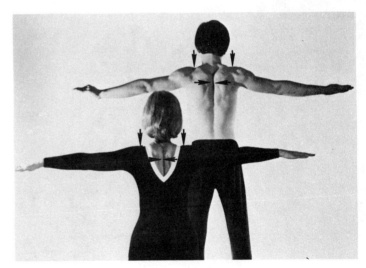

*FIG. 5-2d*

27

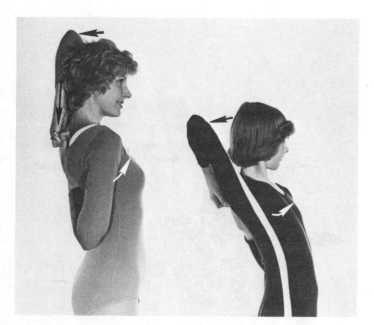

FIG. 5-3a

FIG. 5-3b

## Backward Hand Grip

### TECHNIQUE

1. Sit or stand with a straight spine. Raise your right arm overhead. Bend it at the elbow, bringing your right hand toward your left shoulder. Take your left hand and grab the right elbow. Pull the right elbow directly behind the head, as in **FIG. 5-3a** (left). Keep your head up straight. Your right hand has now been lowered down the center of the spine.

2. Keep hand going down the spine as you bring your left hand down, around, and behind the back, reaching up with it to grasp the right hand, as in **FIG. 5-3a** (right).

3. After you have completed the above correctly, try to pull the right arm and elbow away from the head, as in **FIG. 5-3b** (left). Inhale, elongating, then exhale as you pull the arm further back, as in **FIG. 5-3b** (right). Take 2 more breaths. Remember—the head remains straight. Repeat the same procedure using the left arm.

## Backward Praying Hands

### TECHNIQUE

1. Sit or stand with a straight spine. Place the palms of both hands together behind you at the waist, fingers pointing down, as in **FIG. 5-3c** (left).
2. Turn your fingertips toward the spine and upward, running your hands up your spine, and stopping between your shoulder blades, as in **FIG. 5-3c** (right).
3. Inhale as you raise your sternum and tip your pelvis. Exhale as you shrug your shoulders back, winging your elbows towards the back, as in **FIGS. 5-3d** (left) and **5-3d** (right).
4. Release and repeat this rhythm for 2 more rounds. Release and relax by bending forward and letting your arms drop to the floor in front of you.

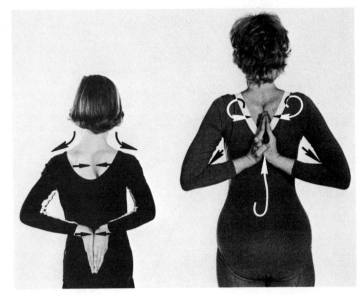

**FIG. 5-3c**

### TIPS

1. If you can not turn your fingers to face up your spine, there is no point in your doing this exercise. Keep working on your Blade Squeeze and Chest Expander Pose.
2. Make sure throughout these two postures that you do not round your shoulders to reach your goal. It is better that you shrug your shoulders back, even if you do not get as far.
3. Try to keep your head straight up even though it will want to lean forward.

### BENEFITS

Releases tension in the shoulders.
Corrects dowager's hump.
Good for arthritic shoulders.

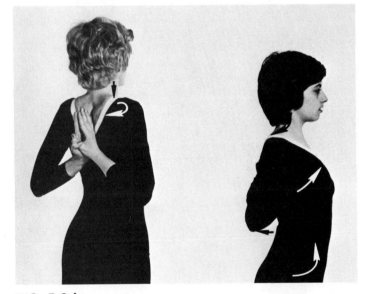

**FIG. 5-3d**

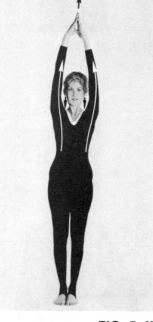

FIG. 5-4a

### TECHNIQUE

1. Stand straight with feet together. Inhale as you raise your arms over head, locking thumbs. Do not arch your back. Tip your pelvis. Exhale as you increase your stretch toward the ceiling, as in **FIG. 5-4a.**

2. Inhale, keeping the extension; lower your shoulders so neck is relaxed, as in **FIG. 5-4b.** Exhale as you reach again toward ceiling, but feel the lift from the forearm and rib cage.

3. Inhale, holding this position, and tighten your buttocks. Exhale as you reach as far as you can to the left without moving your hips, as in **FIG. 5-4c.**

4. In this position, inhale once again as you stretch outward. Now exhale, and you will discover that you can extend your body further and drop lower, as in **FIG. 5-4d.**

5. Inhaling, return to the upright position. Continue the same to the right.

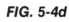

FIG. 5-4b

### TIPS

1. It is very important to concentrate on breathing deeply and smoothly.

2. Notice after each exhalation, when you think you can not go any further, that by inhaling as you elongate and exhaling as you release tension, you *can* bend even further. Throughout this book remember to allow the rhythm of your breathing to ease you into the move. Never force yourself into the move.

3. Keep your head looking forward and do not lean forward or back as you lower to the side with arms and ears staying together. Tighten your buttocks to help keep your hips stationary.

FIG. 5-4d

FIG. 5-4c

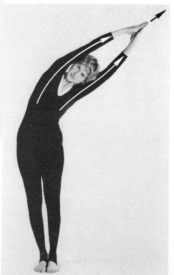

### BENEFITS

Aids bursitis.
Increases lung capacity.
Slims waist and midriff bulge.

# 6 THE CONCAVING AND ELONGATION OF THE SPINE

The average spine is about 27 inches in length. The spine has four normal curves: cervical (neck), thoracic (rib level), lumbar (below the ribs), and sacral (the curve at the top of the buttocks).

The curves of the spine are formed by the different shapes and thicknesses of the individual vertebrae, the discs are cushions of cartilagenous material that separate the individual vertebrae. Any permanent alteration in one curve will affect the curves above or below.

The weight and stress of the entire body passes through each vertebrae. When one overstretches, tugs, or lifts, using his spine in the manner of **DIAGRAM 1,** he is overstraining and putting undue pressure in the lower lumbar area.

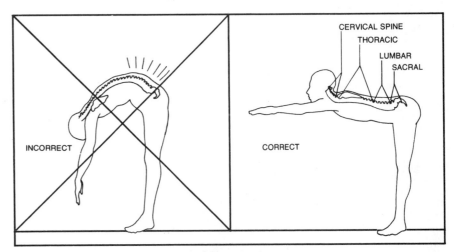

*Diagram 1*

When a disc is damaged or ruptured, a gelatinous matter oozes from it, and severe pain is caused because of the pressure on spinal nerve roots.

The four normal curvatures of the spine allow an optimal operation when stretched or elongated within their range of motion. In teaching students to achieve and maintain a normal spine, I have them work diligently at two basic series of activity. The first, Elongation of the Spine, combines both breath and motion. The student first exhales and pauses briefly, when all the air is expelled so as to pull the abdomen inward and upward toward the backbone at the ribs, while the diaphragm is raised (Tummy-In). Simultaneously with deep, slow inhalation, the shoulders are rotated backward and down so that with this motion and the intake of breath the rib cage is expanded and raised, allowing the sternum to lead the torso upward and forward. Indeed, the direction of "Tummy-In, inhale, and elongate" can be regarded as a single action.

Concaving the Back, the second basic spinal direction found in this series of postures, means stretching the back from head to buttocks so that the spine forms a tunnel (concavity) into which the vertebrae fall and "disappear" instead of standing out as spine-like bumps. You can test for yourself whether you have accomplished "concaving" by running your fingertips up the spinal column, starting just above the sacroiliac.

If you have stretched properly by really "aiming" head and buttocks in opposite directions, your fingers should run in a smooth groove. When this is accomplished, *slightly tip your pelvis forward. Now,* you will feel and experience the elongation in the spine. "Concavity" places the lumbar spine in its natural curve to elongate properly the full spinal column. ((Lest there be confusion, a "concave" back is *not* a sway-back. The concaved back curves inward gently, while the sway-back has a much greater angle of concavity and is to be avoided.

The principle of the elongated, concaved back is basic to many postures, both standing and on the floor, and must be applied until it becomes an automatic, integrated response. Notice its importance in the postures that follow.

## Standing Elongation With Belt

### TECHNIQUE

1. Stand with legs spread 3 feet apart. Clasp your belt as you did in the Chest Expander Pose. Please refer to the Chest Expander Pose for details.
2. Inhaling, elongate as you extend sternum. Exhaling, shrug your shoulders back and down, making a tight shoulder blade squeeze.
3. Inhaling, elongate; tighten your legs by raising kneecaps toward your thighs. Exhale, rotating the hips downward and extending the buttocks toward the back of the room to elongate, as in **FIG. 6-1a** (left).
4. Inhale, elongate, extending your sternum. Exhale, shrugging shoulders back, stretching the arms further down the back as you work to concave the back. With each completed exhalation, do the Tummy-In technique. Just as you inhale, elongate. Keep those kneecaps raised.
5. Take several deep breaths in rhythm with this motion, lowering yourself, as in **FIG. 6-1a** (right).
6. You are leading with your sternum and bending from the hips on the way down. When you are parallel with the floor and your back is concaved, it is very important that you tip your pelvis slightly inward to further elongate the back.
7. While further extending the sternum forward, simultaneously stretch buttocks toward the back of the room. Take several deep breaths in rhythm with this motion. When you have done this, you may come up and relax.

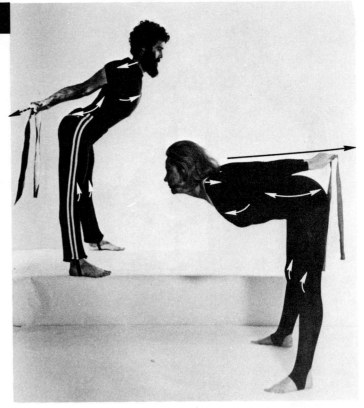

**FIG. 6-1a**

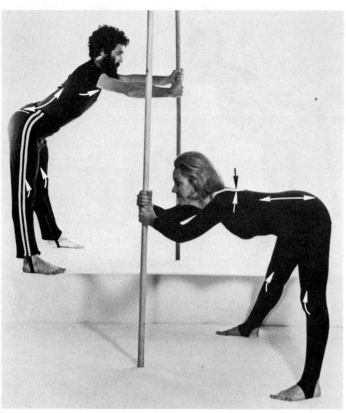

**FIG. 6-1b**

## TECHNIQUE

1. Take hold of a sturdy pole or edge of a doorway with hands at chest level, as in *FIG. 6-1b* (left). Stretch and walk back until your feet are right under your hips.

2. Inhale, then elongate, extending sternum as you raise your kneecaps and extend your buttocks out back as far as you can reach and stretch. Extending your chin, head up, exhale as you rotate the hip downward, extending the buttocks toward the back of the room. Concave the spine, one vertebra at a time, starting from the coccyx bone, working up the back into a shoulder blade squeeze.

3. Take one hand away from the pole and feel the spine. If you are concaving correctly, you should not feel the vertebrae. The "bumps" will disappear. If not, do not lower your hands, but return them to the pole, chest high. Do not lower your shoulders until you feel the lower back is concave.

4. Take 3–5 breaths, working yourself into this elongation stretch as you further concave back while lowering your hands until they are level with your hips, as in *FIG. 6-1b* (right). With each completed exhalation, pull the tummy in and up as you elongate while inhaling.

5. Inhale, then elongate, extending your sternum; exhale as you stretch and reach back with your buttocks while achieving a concave spine.

6. When you have fully concaved the spine, tip your pelvis slightly inward to elongate the back. Further extend the sternum forward and, with buttocks pulling in opposite direction, take several deep breaths in rhythm with this motion. Then slowly come out of it, feeling two inches taller and slimmer.

## Standing Elongation With Counter Top*

1. Apply the same technique as above, but cross your arms. Place the side of your elbow on the counter top, as in **FIG. 6-1c.** Proceed with the Steps 2–6, creating a tight shoulder blade squeeze. Remember to keep kneecaps raised.

## Standing Elongation With Chair

1. Kneel in front of a chair and cross your arms, resting the side of your elbows on the seat. Stretching the back and extending the buttocks back as far as you can, adjust your knees so they come directly under your hips, as in **FIG. 6-1d.** Now proceed as in Steps 5 and 6 of the Standing Elongation with Pole.

### TIPS

1. You must start recessing your spine from the coccyx bone, going from there up the back one vertebra at a time until you work into the shoulder blade squeeze. Do not advance the concaving up the back until you feel the lower back definitely concaved. The spine will "disappear" into the body. I do not mean for you to just drop the back and create a back bend. There is definitely an elongation of the whole spinal column from the extended sternum and buttocks pulling in opposite directions. *When you have concaved, the tipping inward of the pelvis is very important to increase the elongation.*

2. Make sure you keep your knees raised, as in FIGS. 6-1a, b, and c. This helps you to rotate the hips downward and extend the buttocks.

3. Once you accomplish the first step in each variation and have a good concaved lower back, bring your head down so that the ears are lined up with your arms. There is no tension in the neck.

### BENEFITS

A complete stretch to the whole spinal column.
Tones the abdomen.
Works the shoulder region.

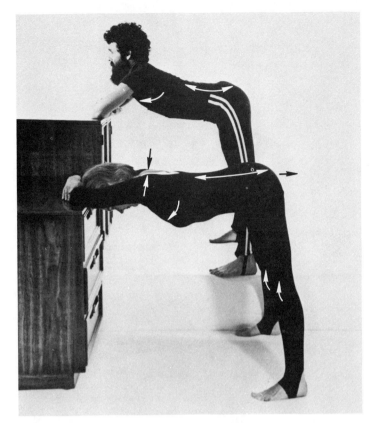

**FIG. 6-1c**

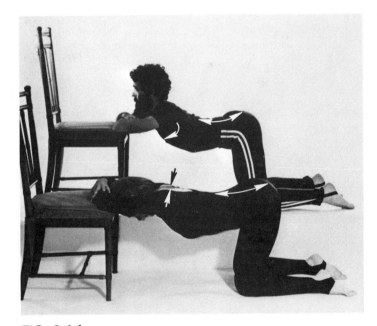

**FIG. 6-1d**

*(Furniture in photographs courtesy of Leone's/Methuen, Ma.)*

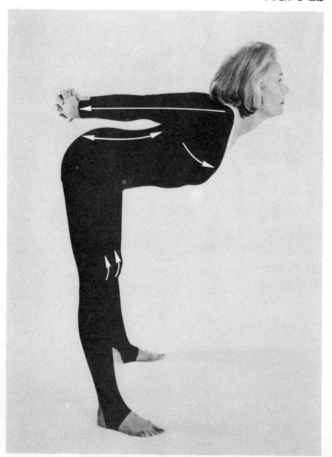

**FIG. 6-2a**

**FIG. 6-2b**

## Basic Warm-Up

### TECHNIQUE

1. Stand straight with feet 3 feet apart and bend forward. Place your hand on the back at the spine. Inhaling, raise your kneecaps, extend the sternum, and rotate your hips as you open the buttocks. Exhale as you work from the coccyx bone, lowering your back down one vertebra at a time. To elongate and maintain balance, keep extending the buttocks toward the back of the room. This will also enhance the concave in the back.

2. Keep your chin up and feel the spine disappear as you inhale, extending the sternum. Then exhale while elongating and concaving the spine further, as in *FIG. 6-2a.* Continue this breathing rhythm for 3 more rounds. Do not forget to keep those kneecaps raised.

3. Now clasp your hands, while shrugging your shoulders back and squeezing blades together. Then reach while hands are still clasped with palms together just beyond your buttocks, as in *FIG. 6-2b.*

4. Inhaling, extend your sternum, raise your kneecaps and rotate your hips. Exhale as you shrug your shoulders back, elongating the spine, and at the same time extend buttocks in the direction of the other side of the room. Continue this rhythmic breathing pattern for 3 more breaths. Do not proceed if you can still feel the bumps of your spine, but repeat.

## Different Hand Positions

### TECHNIQUE

1. To extend this stretch, continue your inhalation procedure, but on the exhalation keep your shoulders back and raise your arms and hands toward the ceiling, as in **FIG. 6-2c.** Continue to elongate the spine by extending the buttocks in the direction of the other side of the room.

2. Apply the basic warm-up technique to get the proper alignment of back and legs. In this variation, lightly interlace your fingers, placing them on the back of the head and keep arms parallel with floor, as in **FIG. 6-2d** (left). Continue with Step 4, p. 36.

3. Repeat as above but fold your arms, holding opposite hands on arms just above the elbows. Keep your arms in line with your ears and do not drop your head. Continue the rhythmic breathing as you extend the arms even further away from the top of your head, as in **FIG. 6-2d** (right). Free the shoulders and be careful that tension doesn't come into the neck.

### TIPS

1. I cannot emphasize enough the importance of the raised knees, the rotation of the hip working the spine inward from the coccyx bone up, extending the buttocks outward, and last, but certainly not least, the leading with the sternum to get full benefits from this posture.

2. Do not proceed into the different arm positions unless you have mastered FIGS. 6-2a and 6-2b.

3. Once you have achieved your recessed spine, tighten your pelvis to further elongate your spine. This move is important for the student with a bad back.

### BENEFITS

Stretches the hamstrings
Elongates the back.
Massages the shoulders.

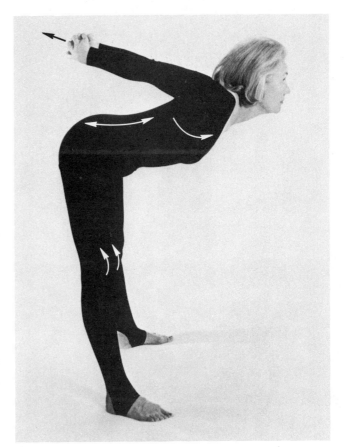

FIG. 6-2c

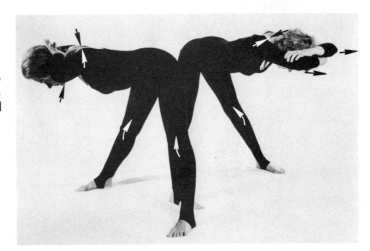

FIG. 6-2d

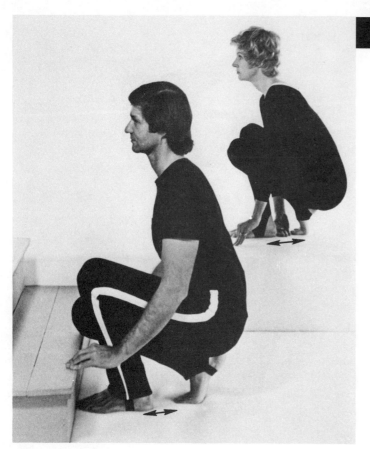

FIG. 6-3a

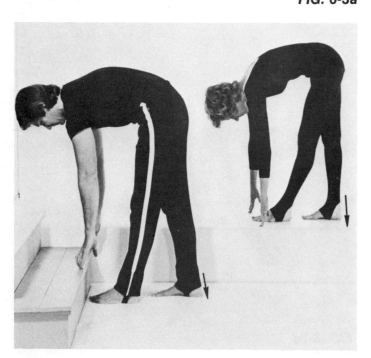

FIG. 6-3b

## TECHNIQUE

1. For those of you who have difficulty touching the floor, please go to the stairs in your home.
2. Stand with your feet side by side up against the step. Now slide the right foot about 3 inches past the left foot but directly in back of its original position, as in walking position.
3. Squat down raising your right heel. To check your correct distance, place your hand between the left heel and right toes. Notice that is what I am doing in **FIG. 6-3a** (right). Now place your fingers at the edge of the step or in line with your toes, as in **FIG. 6-3b** (left).
4. Inhale in this position. Exhale as you come up to straighten the legs, as in **FIG. 6-3b** (left or right). Notice the hunch back. We will be correcting this.
5. Inhale as you raise the kneecaps, concave the spine, do your Tummy-In and elongate to get the full

stretch, as in *FIG. 6-3c* (left or right). Exhale as you work to lower the palms down, as in *FIG. 6-3d.* Do not hunch your back to do so. Keep elongating.

6. Inhale, then exhale as you bend the legs and resume the squat position.

7. In sum, you inhale in the squat position, exhale coming up, inhale elongating the spine, exhale lowering sternum, inhale and repeat the elongation, and exhale returning to squat position.

8. Repeat this rhythm for 5–10 rounds with the right foot behind you. Then repeat the whole cycle with the right foot in front and the left foot in back.

### TIPS

**1.** For those of you who find it difficult to concave your spine as in FIG. 6-3c (left), walk with your hands up one stair at a time until you find your level. You will feel the back elongate while you are leading with the sternum and squeezing the blades together.

**2.** If you have no difficulty touching the floor, you do not need the stair. Squat down and place the fingers in line with the toes, as in FIG. 6-3d (right). If you can accomplish this, you may do the whole exercise with your palms down throughout.

### BENEFITS

Good for sciatica problems.
Circulation in the legs and feet.
Helps back problems.

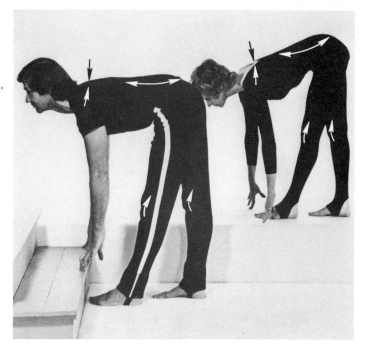

FIG. 6-3c

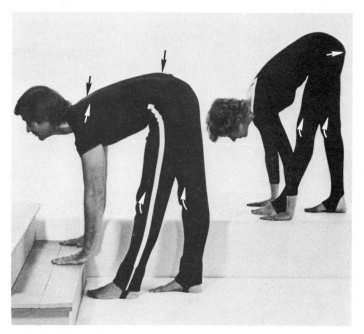

FIG. 6-3d

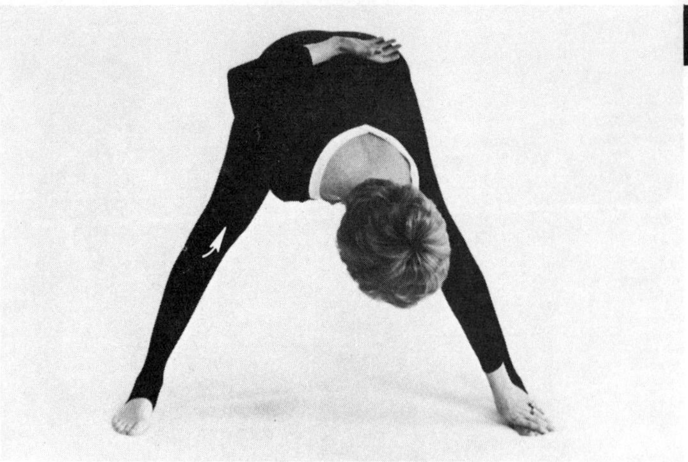

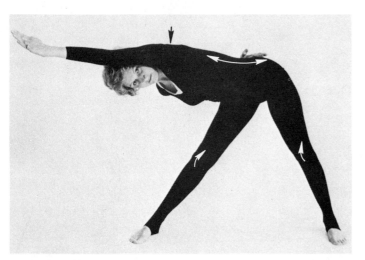

**FIG. 6-4a**

**FIG. 6-4b**

## TECHNIQUE

1. Stand with legs approximately 3 feet apart. Place your right hand at the back of the waist and raise your kneecaps.

2. Inhale, extending the sternum. Raise your left hand up toward the ceiling. Exhale as you bend down reaching out in front, concaving the back. Place your left hand at the left foot, as in **FIG. 6-4a.**

3. Remain concave as you inhale, dragging your left hand to the right foot. Exhale as you reach out and up to waist height, as in **FIG. 6-4b.**

4. Inhale, extend sternum; then exhale, really stretching out, and feeling the elongation from the hip. For a straight extension, keep your arm by your ear and slightly lower your shoulder.

5. Continue reaching outward as you inhale, coming up to a straight position, as in *FIG. 6-4c* (left). Tip your pelvis, tighten your buttocks, keep the reach high as you exhale, leaning back with arm by your ear, as in *FIG. 6-4c* (right).

6. Inhale once again, reaching tall, as in *FIG. 6-4c* (left). Keep knees raised and extend sternum as you exhale, concaving your back and reaching directly out in front, as in *FIG. 6-4d.*

7. Inhaling, feel that elongation in the spine. Exhale as you lower both hands outward and toward the floor. Swing them back and forth, trying to reach as low as possible, relaxing the arms, neck and shoulders but keeping the back concaved. For you more flexible people, hold on to your elbows as you swing.

8. Take several deep breaths in rhythm with the motions. Repeat, starting with the right hand to the right foot.

*TIPS*

1. Really try to stretch beyond your reach all through this posture so you will reach the ultimate stretch and benefits.

2. Throughout this posture, concentrate on keeping the right shoulder down and not letting tension come into the left shoulder. Instead feel the stretch from the rib cage. Do not hunch up—keep shoulders back.

3. In Step 5, it is not how far back you bend, but the elongation of the spine and the stretch of the arm that is important.

*BENEFITS*

Very good for bursitis.
Strengthens the whole back and shoulder region.
Improves posture.
Relieves tension.
Increases energy.

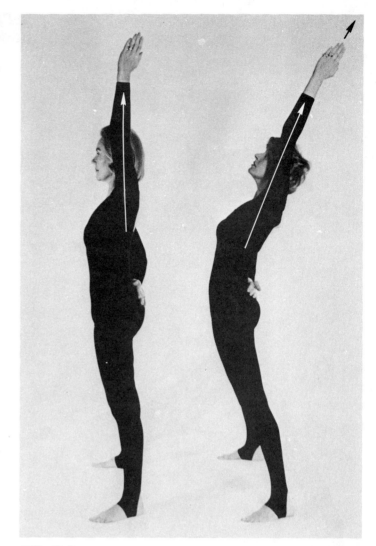

FIG. 6-4c

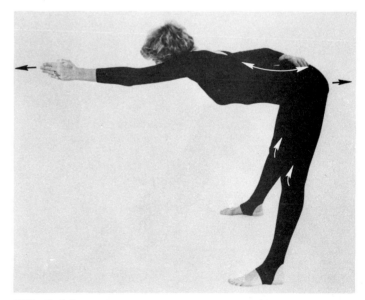

FIG. 6-4d

41

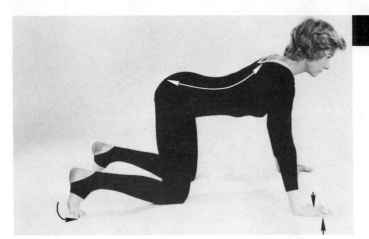

FIG. 6-5a

## Tent Pose

### TECHNIQUE

1. Kneel with your knees and legs hip-distance apart, wrists directly under shoulders. Thighs and arms are perpendicular and your spine is parallel with the floor, as in *FIG. 6-5a.* Note the hand position.

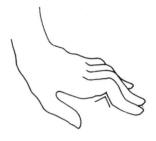

2. Curling your toes under, inhale as you raise your hips high, lifting yourself up high onto your toes. Exhale, raising your kneecaps, and dropping your heels down. Apply Tummy-In, inhale as you look up, and work to concave your spine, as in *FIG. 6-5b.*

3. Exhale as you push with the palms of your hands onto the floor. Take 3 breaths in this position. With each inhalation feel the stretch up the straight legs. As you exhale, work to further concave the spine, making a tight shoulder blade squeeze, bringing your ear in line with your arms, as in *FIG. 6-5c.*

4. If you can master the above with the proper lean in the back, heels down and tummy in, and a good blade squeeze, you may proceed.

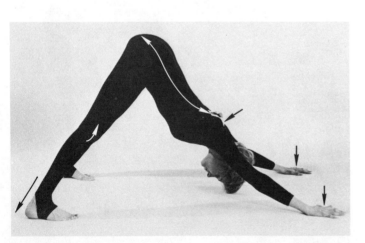

FIG. 6-5b

FIG. 6-5c

## Standing Split Pose

### TECHNIQUE

1. Kneel as in **FIG. 6-5a,** but with your feet and knees together. Inhale, raising your hips high and go way up on your toes. Exhale as you lean in, lowering your heels to the floor. Tighten both by pulling up the kneecaps.

2. Inhale as you raise the right leg up as in **FIG. 6-5d.** Exhale as you lean further into the move, reaching high with the left leg, with heel extended. Take several deep breaths in rhythm with spinal elongation and then lean further into the stretch, bringing forehead toward the floor.

3. Inhale as you bring the left leg down to the floor and resume your kneeling position, as in **FIG. 6-5a,** but with feet and knees together. Repeat Steps 1, 2 and 3, raising the left leg.

### TIPS

1. If you have difficulty in concaving the back, put your hands farther out in front.

2. Do not grip your finger tips into your mat so much that the palm of the hand lifts off from the floor. The correct way is to flatten knuckles nearest the nail so that the pads of your fingers are placed firmly onto the floor. Your second knuckles are bent upward forming an inverted "V" between nail pads and palms, thus pressing the whole palm onto the floor. You now have proper leverage so that your hands will not slide.

3. If you have trouble keeping your heels down, put them up against a wall. Keep hips high, make a strong blade squeeze, and keep arms straight. These are the secrets for getting the right leverage for all the above moves.

4. After you have mastered this technique with heels flat, step back so that it will always be a challenge to work the heels down.

### BENEFITS

Tones the arms, waist, hips and thighs.
Flexibility in the shoulders.
Strengthens the abdomen and wrists.

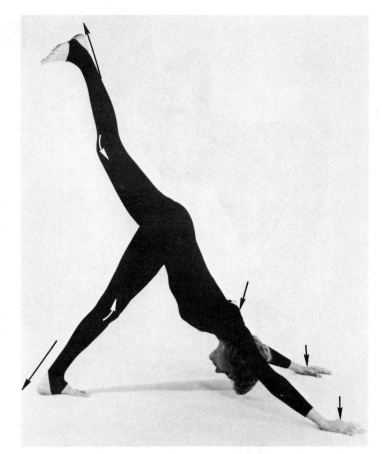

**FIG. 6-5d**

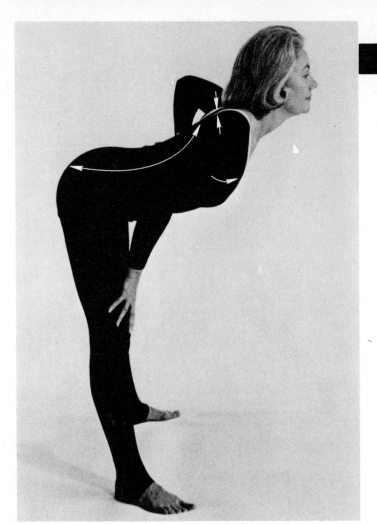

FIG. 6-6a

## Split: Concave Back

### TECHNIQUE

1. Stand with hands on the hips and spread the legs 3–4 feet apart.

2. Inhale; tighten the legs by drawing up the kneecaps. Exhale as you bend forward, leading with the sternum, maintaining a concave back and checking with your hand, as in *FIG. 6-6a.* Let your buttocks aim in the direction of the back of the room.

3. Inhale as you extend further, keeping your body parallel to the floor. Exhaling, apply the Tummy-In technique as you place your fingers on the floor. If you lose the concave stretch in your back, place your hands on a step or stool, as in *FIG. 6-6b.* Work from this point, bending out elbows until you create a shoulder blade squeeze. Now you have achieved the proper back position and can proceed.

FIG. 6-6b

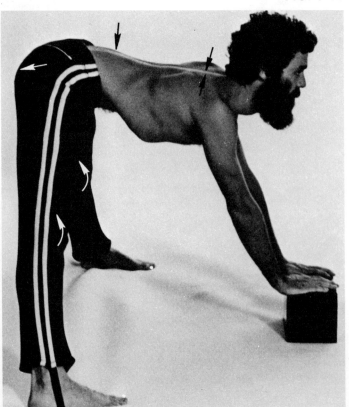

## Split: Elbows Down

### TECHNIQUE

1. Intermediate students should check knees as they inhale and backs as they exhale. Exhaling, perform the Tummy-In, and bend your elbows down on the floor (between the feet), as in *FIG. 6-6c*.

## Split: Hands Through

### TECHNIQUE

1. Advanced Students: inhale as you place your hands through your legs toward the back, as in *FIG. 6-6d*.
2. Exhale as you rest the crown of your head on the floor, keeping the weight of the body on the legs. Do not rest body weight on the head. It helps balance if you tilt the buttocks backward and keep pressure under the ball of the foot.
3. Keep breathing in rhythm while lowering your body even further for 3 breaths.
4. Inhale, raise the head from the floor, and then return hands under shoulders. Keep the head up by making the back concave, as in *FIG. 6-6b*.
5. Exhale as you continue to come up, as in *FIG. 6-6a*.

### TIPS

1. It is very important to proper hip action to keep the legs tightened by keeping the kneecaps raised toward the thigh.
2. After each completed exhalation, do the Tummy-In and up as you elongate.
3. Again, it is not how far down you go into the move that counts but that what you do is done correctly, keeping your spine recessed and checking at each stage.

### BENEFITS

An excellent stretch for the hamstrings and legs.
Increases digestive power.
Elongates the spine.

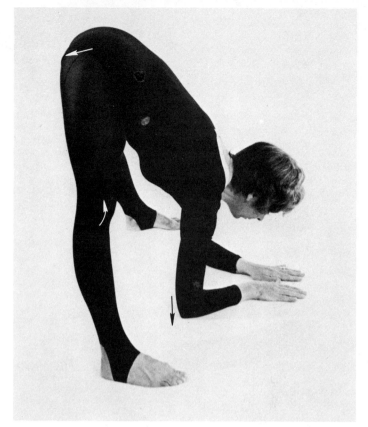

**FIG. 6-6c**

**FIG. 6-6d**

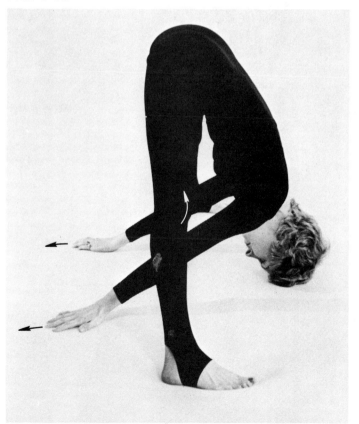

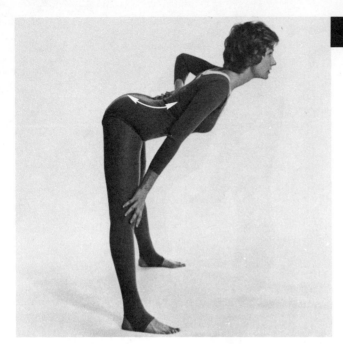

FIG. 6-7a

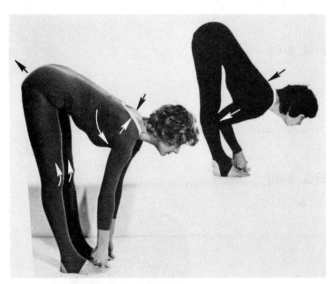

FIG. 6-7b

### Elongating Back

#### TECHNIQUE

1. Stand, spread your legs 3 feet apart as in **FIG. 6-7a.** This will help you warm up. Place hands at the waist with fingertips feeling the spine. Bend forward so your spine will be parallel to the floor. Keeping your chin up, raise your kneecaps and rotate your hips downward. Repeat the above with feet 6 inches apart.

2. Now, you are ready to inhale as you extend your sternum forward, increasing the rotation in the hips. Exhaling, concave the lower back, dropping one vertebra at a time, starting from the coccyx bone and going up the spine. With your fingers, feel the spine move inward and disappear, then slightly tip your pelvis forward.

3. Repeat Step 2 for 3 complete breaths, increasing the elongation with each breath. To aid in the stretch and balance, extend your buttocks in the direction of the other side of the room as you further concave the spine.

4. Please make sure you understand the above elongating exercise and have incorporated each technical move. I cannot stress this enough. If you have not mastered the above correctly, I do not want you to proceed because you will only be straining yourself.

### Pulling From the Big Toes

#### TECHNIQUE

1. From the above position, keep the back concaved and exhale as you bend down to hold the big toes between the thumbs and first two fingers, so that the palms face each other. Hold toes tight, as in **FIG. 6-7b** (left).

2. Keeping your head up, tummy in, inhale, leading with your sternum—not stretching down from the shoulders. When exhaling, shrug your shoulders back, and work your shoulder blades closer together. Keep the kneecaps raised and the back concaved.

3. Inhale again, extending the sternum, and exhale as you shrug the shoulders back and away from the ears while pulling on the toes, which remain on the floor.

4. Now, inhale and elongate again. Exhale as you bend the elbows, as in **FIG. 6-7b** (right). Keep the shoulders shrugged back and free from the neck. Remain in the

position for three or four rhythmic breaths, increasing the elongation with each breath, applying the Tummy-In technique.

5. Inhaling, come up to the position of **FIG. 6-7b** (left). Release the toes and stand up.

## Standing On One's Hands

### TECHNIQUE

1. Apply the technique of **FIG. 6-7a** until you feel you are warmed up enough. Exhale, bend forward and insert your hands under the feet so that the palms touch the soles, as in **FIG. 6-7c** (left).

2. Inhale as you elongate further into the stretch, keeping kneecaps up and working to concave the back by applying the Tummy-In technique after each exhalation.

3. Now, exhale as you bend the elbows, gaining your leverage by pulling upward against the feet. The feet still remain flat on the palms, as in **FIG. 6-7c** (right). Maintain this position for two or three rhythmic breaths. Inhale as you raise up to standing position.

## Palms Down and Facing Back

### TECHNIQUE

1. Please notice the preparation that I have described above for these Standing Forward Bends.

2. Work yourself down into **FIG. 6-7d** (left) with palms on the floor beside the feet, with elbows slightly bent. If you are agile enough, place your hands behind the heels, as in **FIG. 6-7d** (right). Do not bend the legs at the knees, but keep the kneecaps raised. Maintain this position for three breaths and then return to **FIG. 6-7d** (left), while inhaling up to a standing position.

### TIPS

1. If you have difficulty concaving the spine (did not disappear under your finger tips), there is no point in your attempting any of the other positions. Just work on FIG. 6-7a, and in time you will advance.

2. Notice that in FIG. 6-7b (right), 6-7c (right) and 6-7d (left) you are working to get your ribs and chest against the thighs in the beginning. (For more agile students: after your ribs and chest are against the thighs, you may bring the head down, as in FIG. 6-7d (right).

3. I know you want to bend your knees, but if you do, you will not get the full benefit. You just cheat yourself.

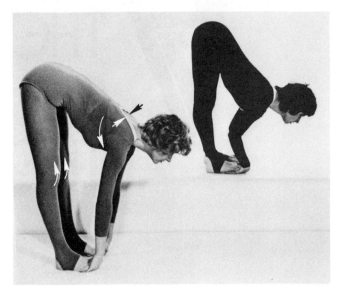

FIG. 6-7c

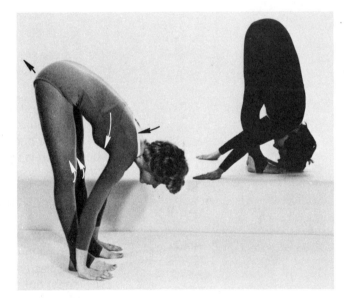

FIG. 6-7d

4. Herniated discs can be greatly helped by the elongating concave back position shown in FIG. 6-7a. If, however, you do not apply this entire technique including a slight tipping of the pelvis, but pull only the head to the knee, you will greatly aggravate the disc problem. You should only go as far as FIG. 6-7a and then practice Standing Elongation With Props and Elongating Legs and Back.

### BENEFITS

Tones the abdominal organs.
Relieves bloating sensation and gastric troubles.
Removes stiffness in the shoulders.
Corrects any minor deformities in the legs.

# 7 THE MUSCLES OF THE LEG

Leg muscles, like all body muscles, consist chiefly of collections of fibrils, which are grouped together to form muscle fibers. Fascia surround the various organs of the body. These bursa act as water cushions to prevent tissue from rubbing or bruising when inflamed. Such inflammations result in pain, swelling, and immobility and are called "bursitis." ("Housemaid's knee" and "tennis elbow" are familiar terms for bursitis.)

Sudden spasmodic and involuntary contractions of muscle fibers produce cramps that can be exceedingly violent and painful.

The skeletal muscles are attached to the bones and are "voluntary," controlled by the will. (Remember: *you* control your body, do not let *it* control you.) Muscles are "exercised" by alternately stretching and contracting them, allowing for optimum blood circulation as well as muscular development and flexibility. In Hatha Yoga, exercise is smooth and flowing.

The following series of postures concern proper use of the bones, joints, and muscles of the legs. The hip and knee joints are among the body's most important because of their use in all activity from simple walking to all lively sports. Good hip and knee joints are essential to good posture. By exercising these muscles properly, you not only gain strength and flexibility in the legs themselves but also strengthen the muscles of the abdomen and lower back.

The hamstring complex and the body's strongest and thickest tendon —the Achilles—are areas where much of our effort will be concentrated. The Achilles is responsible for the plantar flexion of the heel and pointing of the foot. The gastrocnemius determines the shape of the calf and alignment of the whole leg and body because of its relation to the back of the knee. Many of us are aware of these important components in a negative fashion—when years of abuse from wearing high heels, using the legs in a jerky manner, or exercising strenuously without proper relaxation have resulted in a painful "charley horse" or knotted calves.

As you can see in **DIAGRAM 1,** the poor position of the leg brings a lack of body tone in the whole body and creates a strain in the lower lumbar and upper cervical areas.

The corrected posture **(DIAGRAM 2)** shows the pelvis tipped, tummy in, spine flat, neck relaxed, and leg balanced.

**Diagram 1**

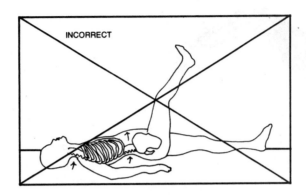

**Diagram 2**

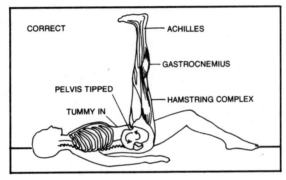

With an understanding of anatomy and placement in mind, the student learns to be aware—to feel—the correct position within a given posture, so that efficient, correct muscular development also becomes a process of learning about both the intensity of muscular action and which muscles to relax when maintaining the activity of others.

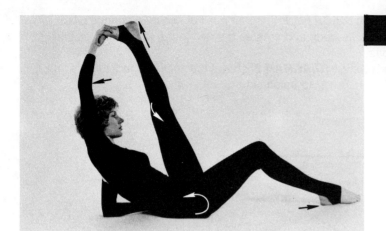

**FIG. 7-1a**

### Leg Raises Warm-Ups

*TECHNIQUE*

1. Lean back up on your left elbow. Bend the right leg to aid you in tipping your pelvis when you push with the heel.
2. Bend left knee to the chest. Place the toes at the wrist of the right hand, which will bring the fingers around the ball of the foot.
3. Inhale, then exhale as you straighten out the left leg, raising kneecap toward the thigh, as in *FIG. 7-1a.*
4. Inhale, extending the heel. Exhaling, contract the abdomen, working the straight leg closer toward you.
5. Repeat Step 4 and on exhalation remember to tip your pelvis further by pushing with your right foot and apply the Tummy-In technique after each exhalation.
6. Maintain the leg close to the face as you let go and slowly lower the leg, leading with the extended heel to the floor.

*TIPS*

1. Throughout these moves, I know the leg wants to bend but I am more interested in how straight it is than how close it is.
2. After each exhalation apply the Tummy-In technique and push away with the foot on the floor. Notice the tilt in the hips. Advance the leg forward taking in the tilt, inhale as you elongate the spine, and repeat.
3. Concentrate on stretching the muscles up the back of the leg as you extend the heel. This will eliminate cramps in the front thigh.

## Calf Pull

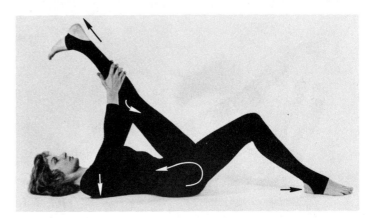

**FIG. 7-1b**

### TECHNIQUE

1. Lie down, bending your knees in order to tip your pelvis. Pressing the small of the back onto the floor, slide your heels down to the point where the back does not come up. Keep both legs at that level so that the knees are even.

2. Inhale as you extend the left heel, and raise the kneecap so that the lower leg leaves the floor to make a straight line with the thigh at the point where the knees are still even. Exhaling, contract the abdomen as you bring the extended leg straight up toward the ceiling.

3. Inhale as you lift the leg further from the hip, but keep the hip on the floor. This will drop the tummy in as the back flattens on the floor.

4. Place your hands gently in back of the leg calf, as in **FIG. 7-1b.** Do it gently—do not squeeze!

5. Now, as you exhale, bring the straight leg closer to your face by bending elbows outward. Do not hunch your shoulders but lower them, keeping the blades on the floor.

6. Keep stretching into this posture by applying the Tummy-In technique first, then inhale as you elongate the leg, pressing heel up. Exhale as you work the leg closer. Do this for 3 breaths. I am more interested in a straight leg than how close it is to your face.

7. I know the knee wants to bend, but concentrate on keeping it straight by raising the kneecap and stretching from the heel. Breathe in, then exhale, while slowly lowering your leg to the floor.

8. Repeat the same to the right side, then once again, on each side.

### TIPS

1. Do not interlock your fingers. Just lightly place all 8 fingers in the center of the calf of the leg. This will give you more flexibility in your arms and shoulders.

2. Make sure your raised leg is completely straight at all times.

3. Advanced Student: this should be done with both legs straight throughout.

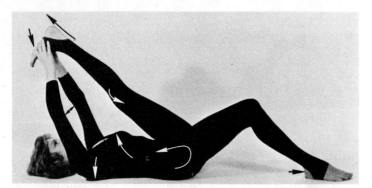

FIG. 7-1c

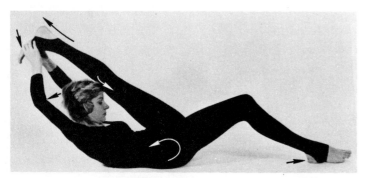

FIG. 7-1d

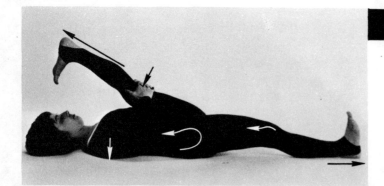

FIG. 7-2a

## Foot Pull

### TECHNIQUE

1. Assume Calf Pull—Step 1 position.
2. Inhale as you bend the left knee to the chest. Place the fingers of both hands around the *ball of the foot* (not the arch—*the ball*).
3. Exhale as you straighten out the left leg, as in **FIG. 7-1c.** Your left knee must be straight to get the benefit of this posture.
4. Keep stretching into this posture by applying the Tummy-In technique, then inhale as you elongate the leg diagonally from the feel and exhale as you work the leg closer. Do this for 3 rhythmic breaths.
5. If you have correctly mastered the above, you may proceed to bring your head to meet the knee, as in **FIG. 7-1d.** Hold for the count of 5 and slowly lower the leg. Repeat the above with the right leg.

### TIPS

1. Make sure the fingers are at the ball of the foot so you are pulling the toes toward the face and extending the heel.
2. The more limber student should do the above posture with both legs completely straight (as the arrows indicate) so as to slide the legs straight.
3. For a variation of FIG. 7-1d, bring the head toward the knee and work your elbows toward the back of the head.

### BENEFITS

Excellent hamstring pull.
Firms and strengthens the abdomen and back muscles.
Good for the shoulder area.

## ADVANCED LEG PULLS

### Hand To Knee Pull

### TECHNIQUE

1. Lie down, bend knees, tip your pelvis and slide your heels down to the point where your back remains on the floor. Keep the right knee bent at that level to start. As you become more flexible, you can straighten out the right leg, as in **FIG. 7-2a.**

2. Inhale and bend the left knee to the chest, interlacing the fingers of both hands at the back of the knee. Exhaling, contract the abdomen, winging out the elbows as you press the knee to the chest. Do not let the knee come up. Tummy-In and inhale as you elongate your torso. Exhale as you work to straighten out the leg, extending the heel as in **FIG. 7-2a.**

3. Keep stretching into this posture by inhaling as you elongate the torso and exhaling as you keep your shoulders to the floor while working the leg straight. Do this for 3 rhythmic breaths.

4. Release the grip and lower the leg. Proceed with the same method, using the right leg.

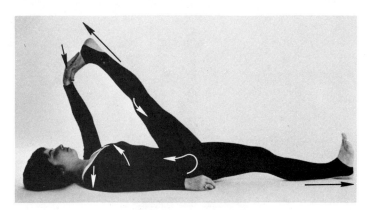

**FIG. 7-2b**

### Toe To Wrist Pull

*TECHNIQUE*

1. While still lying down, inhale and bend the right knee to the chest. Grasp the ball of the right foot with the left hand, with toes at the inside of the wrist. Exhale as you straighten the leg, as in **FIG. 7-2b.** While applying 3–5 rhythmic breaths, bring leg closer to the face if you can, but keep the knee straight. Release the grip and lower the leg slowly. Repeat, using the left leg.

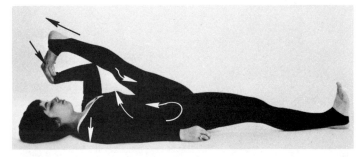

**FIG. 7-2c**

### Elbow To Shin Pull

*TECHNIQUE*

1. Repeat the above Step 1, bending the elbow trying to touch the shin bone, as in **FIG. 7-2c.** Release the grip and lower the leg to the floor. Repeat, using the left leg and right hand.

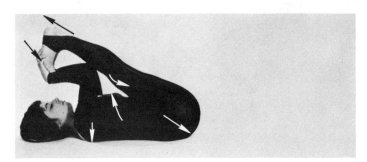

**FIG. 7-2d**

*TIPS*

1. Remember that throughout all these leg raises, the small of the back must remain flat. To accomplish this, keep your pelvis tipped. It helps to reinstate the tip with each exhalation and do the Tummy-In technique before each inhalation.

2. Remember, if this is too difficult, keep the leg on the floor bent.

*BENEFITS*

Excellent for stretching the hamstrings.
Tones and firms the thighs.
Tightens stomach muscles.

### Elbows To Both Shins Pull

*TECHNIQUE*

1. Lying down, inhale as you raise both knees to the chest. Grasp the toes of both feet with both hands so the toes meet the wrists. Straighten out the legs. While applying 3–5 rhythmic breaths, bend both elbows, trying to touch the shin bones, as in **FIG. 7-2d.** Make sure the lower back remains on the floor. Release the grip, slowly lower the legs to the floor, and relax.

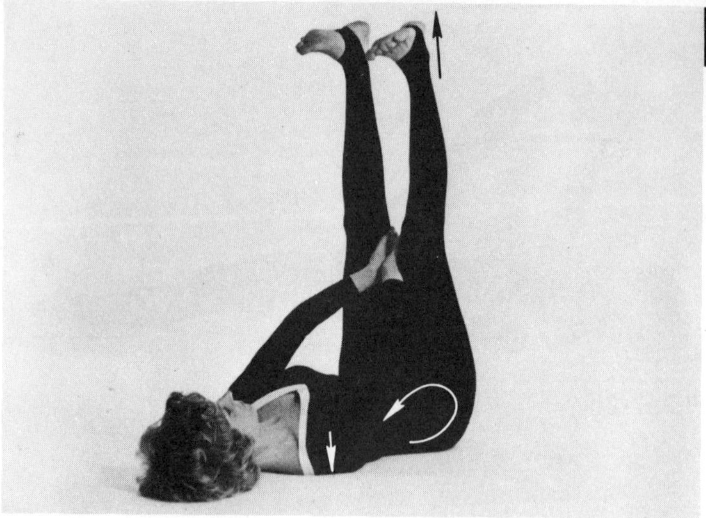

FIG. 7-3a

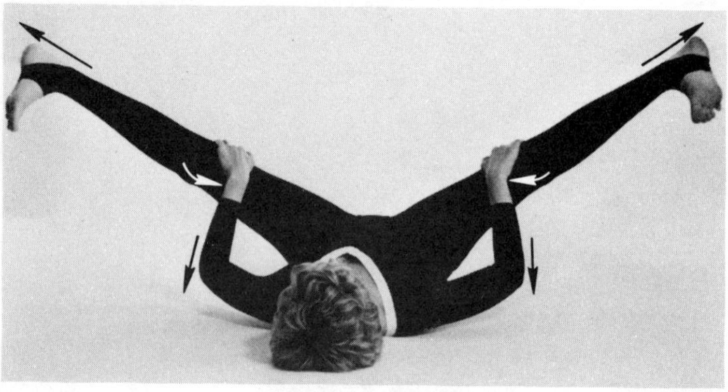

### Warm-Up

*TECHNIQUE*

1. Lie down, bend knees to chest, straighten your legs, bringing heels toward the ceiling.
2. Place your hands between the knees. Inhale, extending your heels, as in *FIG. 7-3a.*
3. Exhaling, split the legs to the sides, keeping the heels extended, as in *FIG. 7-3b.*
4. Tummy-In, inhale, elongate spine as you exhale, applying slight pressure with your hands.
5. Keep the split, let go and exhale as you tip your pelvis, bringing the legs together. Lower the feet to the floor.

FIG. 7-3b

## Hip Balance

### TECHNIQUE

1. Lie down, bend your knees, bring your feet toward your buttocks, open your legs to the sides, tip your pelvis and inhale, elongating torso. Exhale as you raise the left heel toward the ceiling.

2. Place your right hand on your right hip, which remains on the floor at all times. Your left hand is on the inside of the left knee.

3. Tummy-In and inhale as you elongate. Exhale as you lower your right knee out to the side, as in **FIG. 7-3c.** Inhale as you reach tall from the hip with the left leg. Exhale, applying slight pressure with your left hand to lower left leg toward the floor.

4. Concentrate on maintaining your tipped pelvis as you keep the right hip on the floor, while pushing into the floor with the top of your right foot. Do not hunch shoulders. Drop them down to make a slight blade.

5. All this will help balance and hip action as you work, applying 3 rhythmic breaths while lowering the left leg toward the floor, as in **FIG. 7-3d.**

6. To come up, remove the left hand from the leg, inhale, and firmly tip the pelvis. While you exhale, concentrate on a steady leverage at the right hip, as you draw up the left leg. Now bring knees together, sliding feet down to the floor.

7. Repeat to the right side.

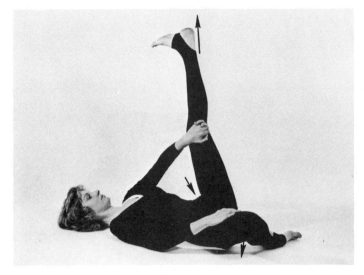

**FIG. 7-3c**

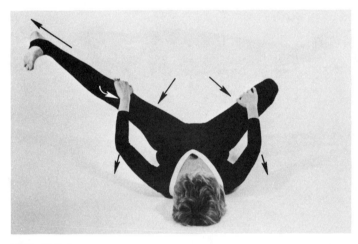

**FIG. 7-3d**

### TIPS

1. Throughout this posture, concentrate on keeping the right shoulder and elbow on the floor.

2. Do not try to get the leg all the way down to the floor. Concentrate on not letting the right hip leave the floor.

### BENEFITS

Loosens the hip.
Tightens the inner thigh.
This is a good diagonal twist.

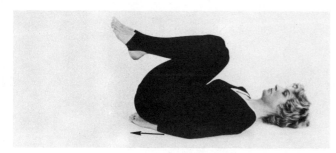

*FIG. 7-4a*

## TECHNIQUE

1. Lie down bending knees to the chest. Clasp your hands (as in **FIG. 7-4a**) under you past the coccyx bone.

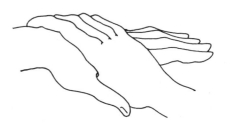

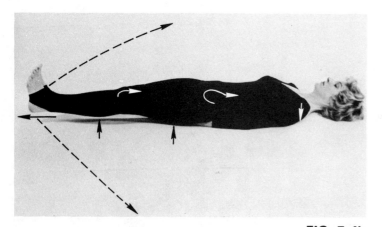

*FIG. 7-4b*

2. You have the right placement if it helps to make the knees hang further over the chest. Make sure that your back is flat on the floor throughout this posture.

3. Lower your legs to the floor. Ease the knees so that you can tip your pelvis as you slide past your hands, removing the hollow in your back.

4. Inhale as you straighten the legs, raise kneecaps, and extend heels at your knee level, as in **FIG. 7-4b.** Retain your breath as you swing your legs apart as far as possible. Exhaling, contract the abdomen as you bring them back to the center, keeping them at the same knee level.

5. Inhale as you raise your legs up to a 45° angle, as in *FIG. 7-4c.* Keeping the lower back flat by tipping, swing legs as wide apart as possible. Exhale as you bring them back to the center (at the same level).

6. Inhale now as you raise your legs to a 90° angle, as in *FIG. 7-4d.* Remember that flat back! Retaining your breath, swing them apart a far as possible. Exhaling, contract the abdomen and bring them back again to the center.

7. Proceed in this same manner, applying the 3 stages on your way down, reversing the breath pattern.

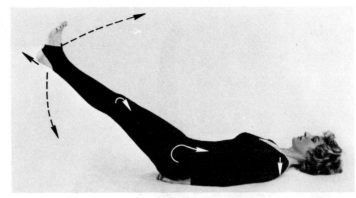

**FIG. 7-4c**

## TIPS

1. It is imperative that the back and tummy remain flat and the pelvis tipped throughout this entire exercise. If you find you are forcing your tummy out for control, this exercise is too hard for you. You should work on developing your abdominal muscles instead.

2. To maintain the proper balance it is important that your hands are in the proper position. Your kneecaps are raised and your heels are extended throughout this whole exercise.

3. When one develops the proper strength in the lower back and abdomen after mastering this exercise, one should accomplish a natural rhythm of breathing in the execution of this posture. With mastery, there is no need to hold the hands under the buttocks.

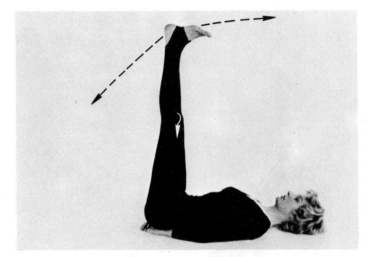

**FIG. 7-4d**

## BENEFITS

Excellent for strengthening the abdomen and lower back.
Firms thighs and hips.
Tightens the buttocks.

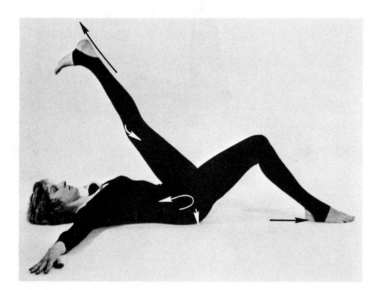

FIG. 7-5a

### TECHNIQUE

1. Lie down with arms stretched out at shoulder level, turning palms down. Bend your knees, tip your pelvis, and slide the heels down to the point just before where your back wants to come up. Reinforce the tip by applying pressure with the right heel onto the floor.

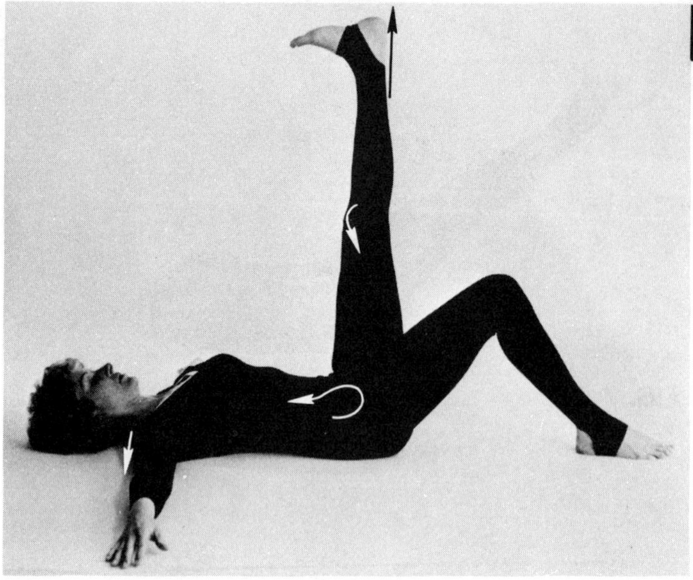

2. Inhale as you raise the left foot up keeping both knees in line. Raise the left kneecap and extend the heel. Exhale as you raise the leg toward the ceiling, as in **FIG. 7-5a.**

3. Inhale as you elongate the left leg up from the hip, using the Tummy-In and up as you maintain leverage by increasing the push of the right heel onto the floor. With this application, exhale while working the leg as close to your face as you can, as in **FIG. 7-5b.** Do not let your buttocks leave the floor. The work is all in the abdomen—the push of the right heel is only an aid.

FIG. 7-5b

4. Keep the left leg at this angle as you inhale to elongate the torso and reinforce the tummy control. Exhaling, contract the abdomen while the leg is still leaning forward, lower the left leg out to the side, working the ankle to cross over the wrist, as in *FIG. 7-5c.*

5. If you can not reach your wrist as in *FIG. 7-5c,* walk over a little to the left with your right heel, still applying pressure. Your left ankle must be at your left wrist in order to continue properly without straining.

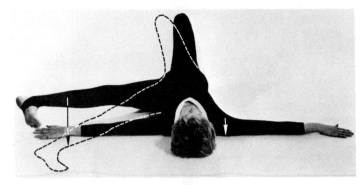

**FIG. 7-5c**

6. Inhale in extreme position, then exhale as you tip even harder so that you will have the proper leverage to bring the foot up from the left wrist and further up as indicated by arrows, continuing to bring the foot smoothly up across the face as in *FIG. 7-5b,* then bring the ankle over to the right wrist, as in *FIG. 7-5d.* If you can not make it, walk the right foot over so your left ankle will definitely cross the right wrist.

7. Inhale in extreme position. Exhale as you tip and bring the leg up from the right wrist, as indicated by arrows, then bring it up smoothly over the face as in *FIG. 7-5b.* Stop when the right foot is directly above the right hip, as in *FIG. 7-5a.*

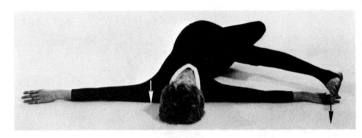

**FIG. 7-5d**

8. Inhale, elongating heel upward, and exhale as you tip and lower the leg to the floor, sliding the right leg to join it.

9. Relax for a moment. I would like to say that you have finished, but there is still your right side to do, so just repeat and reverse the above instructions.

### TIPS

1. Throughout this whole exercise, concentrate on keeping your shoulders down. It will give you leverage.

2. During the pendulum swing from wrist to wrist, make sure you maintain the proper lean and leverage so you will feel it working in the back of the thigh. If it is not felt, you are not doing it correctly.

### BENEFITS

Slims down the waist.
Reduces thighs and hips.
Definitely tones the abdomen.

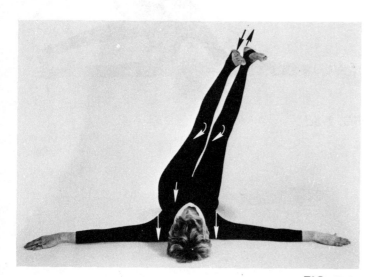

FIG. 7-6a

### TECHNIQUE

1. Lie on the floor with arms stretched out to the sides, shoulders flat on the floor and palms down. Bend the knees to the chest, inhaling as you raise your legs straight up to the ceiling, with kneecaps raised toward the thighs and heels extended, as in **FIG. 7-6a**. Exhale, contract the abdomen as you lower the legs to the halfway point toward the right, as in **FIG. 7-6b**. Check to see that legs are vertical, heels are uneven and your right hip stays on the floor, as in **FIG. 7-6c**. Inhale as you tip your pelvis, exhale, and force the hip further onto the floor. Do this twice. Inhale, pushing the shoulders and elbows on the floor for leverage. Exhale with the abdomen contracted as you raise both legs up toward the ceiling again. Proceed with the same movements to the left side.

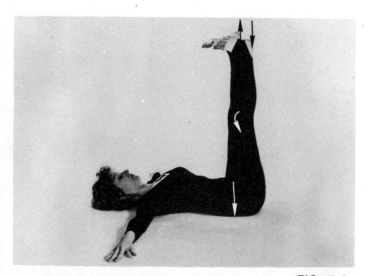

FIG. 7-6b

FIG. 7-6c

60

2. Go through Step 1 again, but this time lower the legs only to the point where you can still maintain the hip leverage, as in *FIG. 7-6d.* Do not go too far and have to sacrifice control of the hip. The angle and approach for lowering the leg is from the hip level, as in *FIG. 7-6c.*

3. Inhale, and then exhaling, bring the legs up, then bend and lower them to the floor.

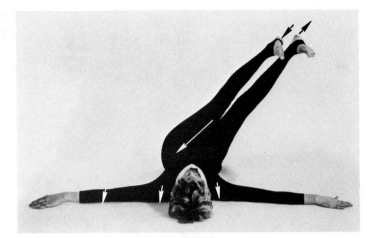

**FIG. 7-6d**

*TIPS*

1. Do not allow elbows and shoulders to leave the floor at any time during this entire posture.
2. Throughout this posture, when your feet are at an angle, the heels must remain *un*even. The heel of the upper leg is at the ankle of the lower leg.
3. In coming up from the side position, make very sure that you are tipped, that your back is down, your shoulders shrugged down, and your tummy is in. If you are unable to apply the technique of keeping your back down and tummy flat, this exercise is too hard for you. Work on the Bent Leg Twist (in my first book).

*BENEFITS*

Excellent for firming and toning the abdominal organs.
Alleviates round shoulders.
When done properly, strengthens the lower back.

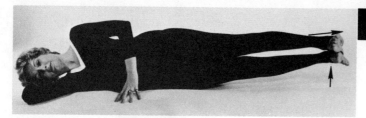

**FIG. 7-7a**

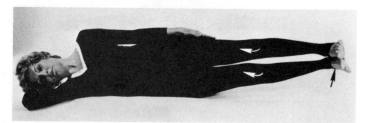

**FIG. 7-7b**

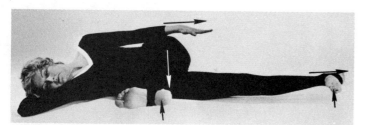

**FIG. 7-7c**

*TECHNIQUE*

1. Lie down on your right side. Bend your right elbow and make a fist with your hand, placing your head on the curled little finger.

2. Align yourself so you are straight from head to heel. You can place your left hand on the floor at your waist for support.

3. Tummy-In, inhale, elongating. Exhale, extend heels and raise both legs from the floor, as in *FIG. 7-7a.* When you have your balance you may place your hand on the thigh, as in *FIG. 7-7b.* Take breaths in this position.

4. From this position, keeping the right leg off the floor, exhale as you bend the left knee up front as far as it will go. Apply the Tummy-In action, flowing into an inhalation.

5. Keeping the left knee at this level, exhale as you work to straighten the leg out in front, as in *FIG. 7-7c.* Hold. Slowly bring the leg back.

6. With both legs off the floor, extend heels. Inhale to elongate. Tighten your buttocks and keep the kneecap facing forward.

7. As you exhale, raise your left leg up toward the ceiling as far as you can.

8. Tighten the buttocks some more so you will not fall backward. Apply the Tummy-In action and flow into an inhalation as you turn the knee to face you. Exhaling, hold on to the leg.

9. Inhaling, extend sternum to elongate. Exhale as you bring the leg closer to your face, as in *FIG. 7-7d*. Keep elongated with buttocks tight so you will not drop your left hip.

10. Take 3 breaths in rhythm with this motion. Slowly lower the leg. Relax on your side by curling up into a ball before repeating on your left side.

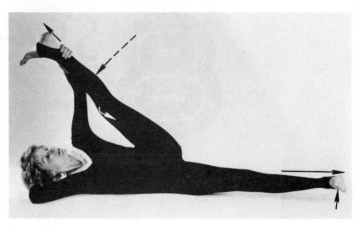

**FIG. 7-7d**

*TIPS*

1. I cannot stress enough the importance of the tightened buttocks to keep you aligned.
2. Make sure you keep the extended heels throughout all steps.
3. In addition to these details, *keep the neck relaxed*.
4. It is helpful to stretch the arm lengthwise along the body, as in FIG. 7-7b and 7-7c, for balance.
5. If you find that you are tired doing all 4 variations in one sequence, you may rest in between.

*BENEFITS*

Firms the hips and thighs.
Tones the abdomen.
Promotes balance.

# 8 STRENGTHENING THE ABDOMINALS

Your lungs and heart are encased in a rib cage and surrounded by muscles. Your stomach, intestines, liver, and kidneys rest in the basin of your pelvic bones; these organs are further confined within a stretchable container that is made up of four muscles: transversalis abdominis, a broad sheet of muscle that lies horizontally around the trunk; internal and external obliques that make a diagonal pattern across the abdomen; and rectus abdominis, the flat muscle that forms the front of the abdomen.

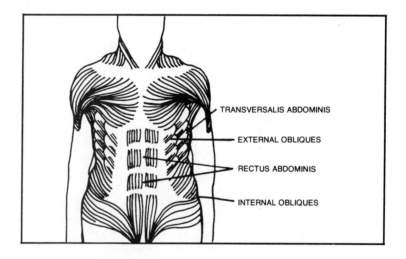

TRANSVERSALIS ABDOMINIS

EXTERNAL OBLIQUES

RECTUS ABDOMINIS

INTERNAL OBLIQUES

The abdominal muscles are the most difficult group to involve in beneficial exercises. These are supportive muscles whose only function is to hold your organs in place, not to move you. They are not designed to swing the body.

Probably the most familiar exercise for toning the abdominal muscles is the Sit-Up. Improperly executed, the Sit-Up does more harm than good, not only to the abdominal muscles but to those in the lower back. Most people approach the Sit-Up with an attitude of psychological defeat—they are tense, with breath held, abdomen pushed out, lower back straining to force the shoulders forward—and end in physical defeat, retaining a hard, protruding "potbelly" abdomen and, possibly, a weakened lower back.

INCORRECT

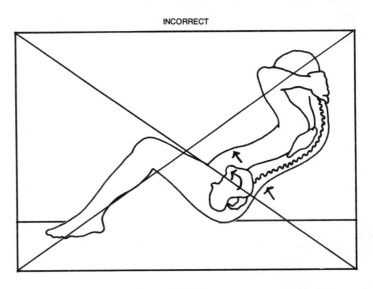

**Diagram 1**

CORRECT

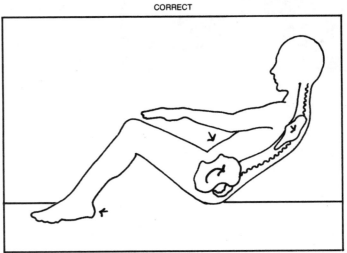

**Diagram 2**

To gain the greatest benefit from exercises to strengthen abdominal muscles, you must concentrate at all times on using these muscles properly to make them work for you. I know it is not easy, but do join me in the following exercise—the Sit-Balance—and experience the correct way to approach the dreaded Sit-Up. You will eventually have a nice, conditioned, *flat* tummy as a result of your effort.

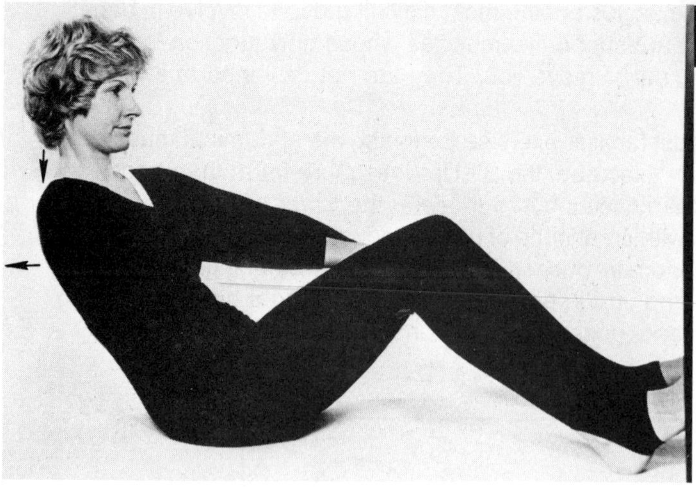

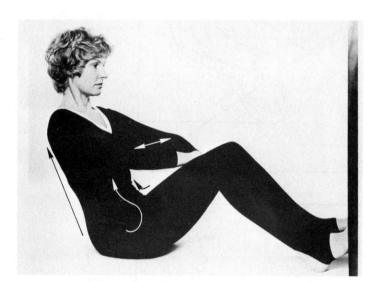

FIG. 8-1a

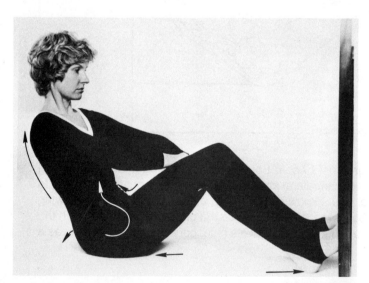

FIG. 8-1b

## TECHNIQUE

1. Sit up, bend your knees and plant the ball of the foot against the wall. Place your hands on the inside of your thighs close to the knees. Pull the inner thighs hard toward you, using them for leverage. This will round, open and widen your shoulder blades. *Do not* hunch them up.

2. Lean back to straighten arms and make sure your tummy is relaxed, as in *FIG. 8-1a.* This is our starting position.

3. Exhaling, contract the abdomen and tip your pelvis, pulling your tummy in and up as you hold your breath.

4. Inhale, elongate, extending your sternum and creating a very slight blade squeeze, as you wing out your elbows *(FIG. 8-1b).* Do not relax the tummy; lift when you elongate.

5. Exhale, maintaining your lift and raised sternum, and push away with your heels. Without moving away, slide your coccyx back along the play in the skin until the slack stops. (Think of the manner in which your skull and scalp move.) You will be lowering the small of your back slightly closer to the floor, as in *FIG. 8-1c.* This is your Balance Point. Make sure you do not slouch; keep the lift and raised sternum.

FIG. 8-1c

6. When you have achieved the proper tipping and control for this balance, without having your tummy pop out, let go of your thighs, as in *FIG. 8-1d.* Keep the back and tummy motionless. It helps to tighten the anal muscles to aid in keeping the tummy in.

7. Hold this position for 3 breaths. With each inhalation, reassess the proper elongation; with each exhalation, reinforce the proper tip in the pelvis and the lift in the tummy.

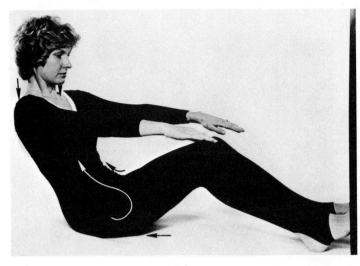

**FIG. 8-1d**

## TIPS

1. Throughout this exercise, apply a very conscientious effort to find and maintain the proper balance. Do not sag, slouch, or completely relax in this exercise.

2. If at any time the tummy pops up, *stop and begin again from the beginning.*

3. There is no reward for going on to the next step if the previous step was done incorrectly. You are in competition with no one except yourself. And you are getting greater value at *your* level of Balance Point than by straining to get further.

## BENEFITS

Flattens and holds in the abdomen.
Trims the waistline.
Eases lower back pressure.

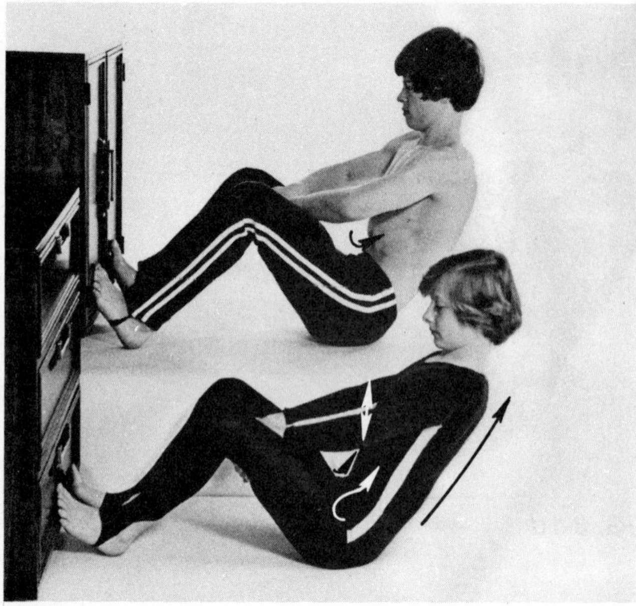

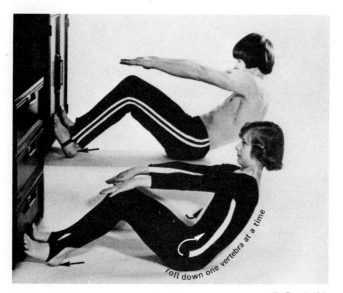

FIG. 8-2a

## Downs

### TECHNIQUE

1. Assume the proper Balance Point of the Sit-Balance (Steps 5 and 6, as in **FIG. 8-2a**).

2. Lightly place hands above the knees, check that your tummy is in, pelvis tipped, spine elongated.

3. Keep the elongation from within the length of the spine and focus your attention on your abdomen, feeling the proper control you have to maintain. Inhale in one long elongated breath, but you exhale in many short forceful releases of that one breath. With each expulsion, your tummy will pull in. Continue to tip your pelvis each time you lower a vertebra to the floor, starting from the coccyx bone. The slower you lower the better.

4. Continue exhaling, pushing with your heel, and let your fingers lightly slide down the thighs, as you slowly continue lowering one vertebra at a time to the floor, as in **FIG. 8-2b.** Then lower your head to the floor.

FIG. 8-2b

## TECHNIQUE

1. You are lying down, hands on the thighs, knees bent, as in **FIG. 8-2c.**
2. Tummy-In, inhaling, elongate from the hip, pressing the back onto the floor.
3. Exhaling, contract the abdomen, raise your head, round your shoulders and work the fingers up the thighs as you push with your feet.
4. Again, there is a change of breathing rhythm. It is not smooth but short, quick expulsions. With each expulsion, there is a further tipping of the pelvis. The result is a series of jerky motions as you roll the spine up from the floor one vertebra at a time.
5. On your way up do not slouch in the midriff, but keep the elongation in the rib cage, as in **FIG. 8-2d.**
6. Bring yourself up to **FIG. 8-2a** and continue this Down and Up motion for five rounds.

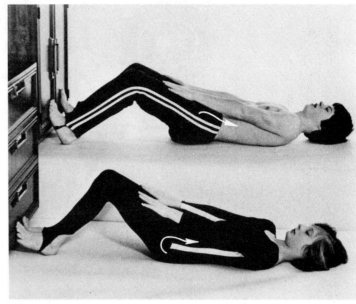

**FIG. 8-2c**

## TIPS

1. It will be very helpful if you concentrate on tightening your anal muscles when rolling down and up. It will help you to control your tummy.
2. Do not accept the idea that your tummy will not pull in. If you have elongated and tipped your pelvis properly, it *will* pull in. The most common mistake is to slouch, thereby closing the space where the tummy should drop in.
3. In lowering and raising your back to and from the floor, it is helpful to push continually with your heels so as to slide the coccyx back along the "play" in the skin. (Remember the scalp?)
4. As you master these exercises, you will do them with a fluid motion, but will maintain the same control.

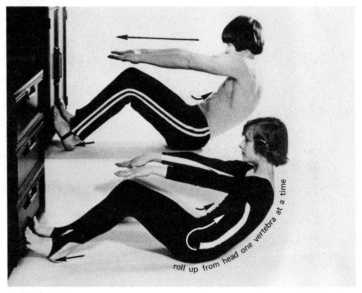

**FIG. 8-2d**

## BENEFITS

Firms and controls the abdomen.
Tightens nature's natural girdle.
Improves your posture.

# 9 THE ALL-INCLUSIVE WARM-UP

The Sun Salutation is an excellent warm-up and toning exercise. The ideal time to practice it is in the morning, but it can be used to invigorate or relax the body at any time.

Insomniacs find it helpful in working out tensions and after 6 rounds, the victim of sleeplessness is usually grateful for a bed.

The Sun Salutation is made up of 12 movements, repeated in a smooth successive manner. The whole muscular structure is brought into play. This exercise is a warm-up and conditions you for the asanas (postures). Along with toning up the muscles, there is a quickening and intensification of the respiration and cardiac rhythm, without induced fatigue or breathlessness. Here we synchronize movement with breathing, and this thoroughly ventilates the lungs. With practice, one gains grace, coordination and confidence and one also prepares the body for any sport.

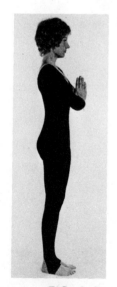

FIG. 9-1a

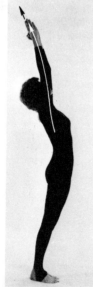

FIG. 9-1b

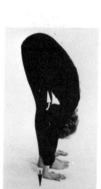

FIG. 9-1c

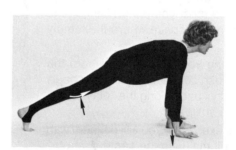

FIG. 9-1d

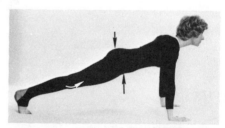

FIG. 9-1e

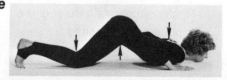

FIG. 9-1f

70

### TECHNIQUE

1. Stand straight with palms together *(FIG. 9-1a)*. Pause for a moment, taking a Complete Breath and bringing calmness to your mind.

2. Inhale as you raise both arms over your head. Tighten buttocks as you lean back *elongating (FIG. 9-1b)*.

3. Exhale and reach out, not bending backwards but concaving the back, then extend downward, keeping your knees straight. Touch the floor with your fingers on the outside of your feet. Your fingers should be in line with your toes and not moved from this position until you raise them for Step 11. Bend the elbows as you lower the ribs and chest to the thighs *(FIG. 9-1c)*.

4. Bend your knees while sliding your right foot as far back as you can. Inhale, and, looking up, keep the left leg vertical as you straighten out the right knee *(FIG. 9-1d)*.

5. Retain your breath, tighten buttocks and slide your left foot back alongside the right foot. You are in a straight incline *(FIG. 9-1e)*.

6. Exhale as you bend knees to the floor; arch back so buttocks are up in the air. Bend the elbows with control from the arms, and slowly lower the chest and face to the floor *(FIG. 9-1f)*.

7. Drag yourself forward until flat on the floor. Relax the feet. Inhale as you raise your forehead, nose, chin, chest, and ribs. The lower part of the body remains on the floor from the navel down. This is called the Cobra posture *(FIG. 9-1g)*.

8. Curl your toes under, raising your hips until your arms and legs are straight. Exhale. Push with the palms of your hands as you lean onto your heels, flattening them against the floor. At the same time, work the head toward the floor, with straight arms *(FIG. 9-1h)*.

9. Shift your weight to the left hand and left foot as you bring the right foot up forward in line with the fingers. Inhale, look up, and straighten out the left knee *(FIG. 9-1i)*.

10. Balance on the fingers as you lift yourself up, bringing the left foot beside the right. Exhale as you place the palms of the hands down on the floor beside the feet. Straighten the leg, bringing ribs and chest down along the legs until the forehead stretches below the knees *(FIG. 9-1j)*.

11. Inhale as you reach out, concaving the spine; then bring your arms up, raising the knees, tighten the buttocks, and look at your fingers *(FIG. 9-1k)*.

12. Exhale as you return to the original standing position, as in *FIG. 9-1l*. Do not rush. Do the steps slowly so that you have time to achieve each posture correctly. Repeat the entire series, stressing the left leg this time. This constitutes one complete round. Four rounds make for a nice warm-up, but you may do as many as you feel necessary.

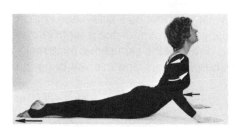

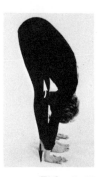

**FIG. 9-1g**

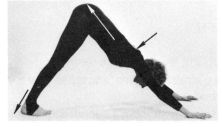

**FIG. 9-1h**

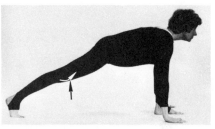

**FIG. 9-1i**

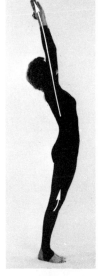

**FIG. 9-1j**

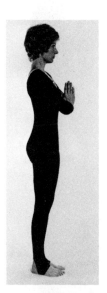

**FIG. 9-1k**

**FIG. 9-1l**

1. The correct way to do these postures is to have the fingers beside and in line with the toes (FIG. 9-1b). The fingers should not leave this position throughout any steps, except the first and last 2 positions.

2. It is more important to get each posture exactly right than to breeze through. Remember this is a warm-up exercise, and we want to work out those little spots that bother all of us.

3. In reference to Step 3, if one is just hanging in this position, without achieving a concave back, then place the hands on the shin bones (while pushing) and this will help elongate the back. Do not pull yourself down—*elongate*—lead yourself down.

4. In reference to Step 4, it is important that you maintain a straight incline while straightening the leg. Keep the bent leg vertical; do not lunge forward.

5. In reference to Step 5, be sure that your feet are back far enough so that the buttocks are not up in the air, the tummy is in, and the back does not arch.

6. In reference to Step 6, I have given you the beginner's approach. Once you master this, proceed further. You are now in the position of FIG. 9-1f. Ease the knees, bend the elbows, arch the buttocks up in the air, as you now slowly, but with control, press the knees, chest and face to the floor—all at the same time.

7. In reference to Step 7, when you are up in the Cobra position, make sure that your elbows are bent and beside your body. Try to make a Blade Squeeze in order to keep your shoulders away from your ears.

8. In reference to Step 8, it is difficult for each student to get the heels flat in this position. The object is to stretch the backs of the legs. If you find it near impossible, you may walk your feet up a little—and I mean "a little!"—so that you can experience a slight lean in getting the heels down. At the same time, try to make a Blade within the shoulders and this will bring the head in closer.

9. In reference to Steps 9–12, these are basically the same as Steps 1–4.

*BENEFITS*

An excellent warming-up exercise.

Limbers, stretches, firms, and tones nearly every part of the body.

An excellent energizer. I cannot say enough for it.

# 10 HEADSTAND

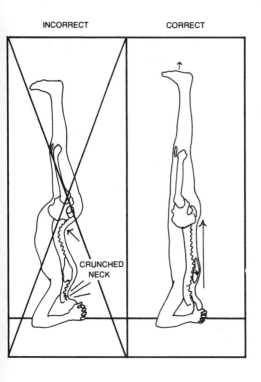

INCORRECT          CORRECT

CRUNCHED NECK

The Yoga Headstand is often referred to as the "King of the Asanas" because of all its beneficial results and the overwhelming sense of satisfaction you will experience on achieving the Headstand.

The position brings perfect upside-down equilibrium. The solid base of support is a triangle formed by the top of the head, forearms, and elbows, which are open at a straight angle.

The difficulties of doing the Headstand are exaggerated by people simply because they are not acquainted with the technique. Many fling their feet wildly into the air, take a tumble, and decide that this is not for them.

The Headstand can be performed by anyone who is endowed with normal physical health, and this posture brings excellent relaxation to all the muscles, since the axis and center of gravity in the body is exactly in the supporting triangle.

The physiological advantages are to be found in a greater flow of blood to the head, bringing an increased blood supply to the endocranial nerve centers, and a discharge of blood and weight from the lower limbs. The increased heart action provides for a better distribution of blood to all parts of the body. Obviously people stricken with chronic heart or vascular diseases should avoid the Headstand. If you have any doubts, check with your physician before trying this or any Yoga postures.

For the student whose balance is either insecure or tilts to the stronger side, it is helpful to use corner walls; this area will help the beginner to keep the Headstand symmetrical.

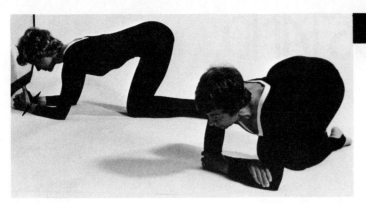

**FIG. 10-1a**

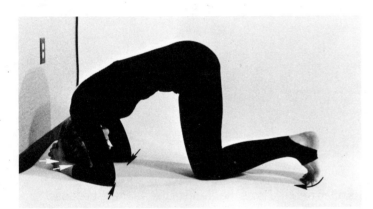

**FIG. 10-1b**

*TECHNIQUE*

1. Crouch down on the floor with elbows and wrists in front of you. To judge how far apart the elbows should be from one another, place the thumbs and index fingers right into the crook of the arm, as the woman on the right in *FIG. 10-1a* is doing. This should be the same distance as the width of your shoulders and is your personal measuring gauge for the proper balance in the Headstand.

2. Make sure that the elbows never wing out any wider. Interlace your fingers with the thumbs pointing up. Apply pressure with the cushions of the fingers onto the knuckles causing a strong grip within the fingers. Palms are not together, as I am doing on the left in *FIG. 10-1a.* Do not get so carried away with making such a strong squeeze that your wrists come off the floor. Turn the wrists inward, pressing them onto the floor and causing a contraction of the muscles of the forearms, upper arms and shoulder blade area. Make note of this feeling and the control it gives you. *It is this control that holds and balances you in the headstand—not just the head or neck.*

3. To put this strength into a warming up exercise for the Headstand, move your knees away from the elbows so that the thighs are straight, as in *FIG. 10-1b.* Place the tip *top* of the head on the mat. If your forehead touches the mat, you are not on the *top* of the head. Now interlace your fingers and cup your hands around the back of the head, as in *Fig. 10-1b.*

4. Curl your toes under and raise the legs from the floor to straighten them, as in **FIG. 10-1c.** Apply that squeeze as in **FIG. 10-1a,** as you push your wrists and forearms onto the floor. This will give you the leverage that you need to raise your head.

5. Push wrists in and down on the floor as you lean back, lifting your shoulders up and back, and working your shoulder blades together. With your head up, bring it back so your nose will be in line with your elbows, as in **FIG. 10-1d.**

6. Hold this position, breathing normally until you feel assured of the proper strength and balance needed to master the Headstand. Come back down, as in **FIG. 10-1b.** Check your personal measuring gauge, as in **FIG. 10-1a** (right), to see that your elbows have not sprung out. Go up again, treating this posture as a ''push-up'' approach for gaining coordination and strength in your arms. Do this 3–5 times if you are doing only this exercise. For those of you who plan to do the Classic Headstand, do the Warm-Up only once or twice for preparation.

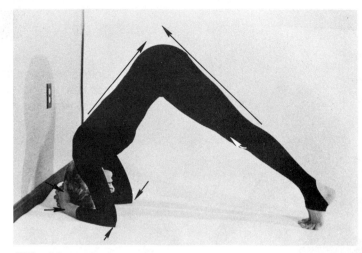

**FIG. 10-1c**

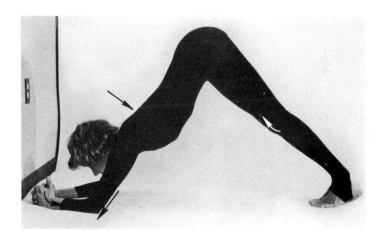

**FIG. 10-1d**

*TIPS*

**1.** The leverage one uses in this warming-up exercise and the Classic Headstand comes not so much from the gripping effect of the fingers as from pushing of wrists, forearms, and elbows directly down onto the floor. Make sure that you do not misunderstand the above. You do *not* receive your strength from winging out the elbows, which can be corrected if it occurs (when you check your personal measuring gauge on coming down to kneeling position).

**2.** Make sure that you keep the legs straight.

**3.** Do not put any tension in the neck.

**4.** Please be meticulous about reading these instructions. They are all very important in accomplishing the Headstand.

*BENEFITS*

Strengthens and tones the wrists, arms and shoulders.

Develops coordination and control.

Promotes self-confidence for the Headstand.

Unless you have accomplished the Headstand Warm-Up correctly, please do not discourage yourself by trying to accomplish the Classic Headstand. Those who are ready may begin.

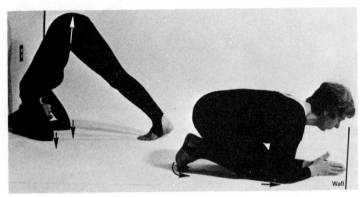

FIG. 10-2a

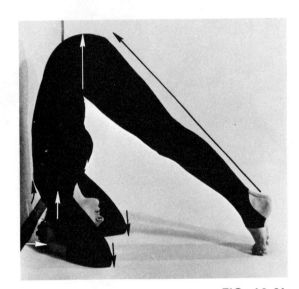

FIG. 10-2b

FIG. 10-2c

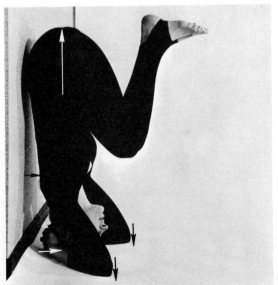
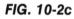

*TECHNIQUE*

1. Kneel down on the floor. Judge your elbow distance by using your personal gauge. With your knees right against the elbow, place your palms together, finger tips to the wall, as in *FIG. 10-2a.* Interlace your fingers, adjusting yourself so you are only three inches away from the wall. Now, interlace your fingers with thumbs pointing up, place top of your head on the floor, cupping your hand around the back of the head, leaving about an inch between the little finger and floor. If you start this way it will keep your fingers from all being under the head. Make sure that knees are in line with your elbows. Tuck your toes under, as in *FIG. 10-2a* (right).

2. Straighten the legs, as in *FIG. 10-2a* (left), keeping the toes where they are, as in *FIG. 10-2a* (right). Do not slide toes back.

3. Tilt back until you are on your toes, as in *FIG. 10-2b.* Do not collapse. Maintain the effort you are applying onto the floor with your elbows and wrist, keeping a lift in your shoulders. Do not let yourself just drop onto the wall. Lift high from the hips as you tilt, trying not to touch the wall. This puts your hips in the proper balancing position for the next step.

4. If you have leaned far enough, you will note that your knees automatically want to bend toward the body. Do not kick up. You simply bring one knee at a time toward the chest, as in *FIG. 10-2c.*

5. Using the strength in your arms, elbows, wrist and hand grip, raise your thighs by bringing your feet

directly above your spine, as in **FIG. 10-2d.** So you will know that your feet are in line with your spine, gently bring *one* toe to the wall. Touch just your toe, not your heel (heel touching will merely cause you to drop back onto the wall). Try to maintain control away from the wall. Hold.

6. Do not proceed further unless you can hold this position in balance, and without an arch in your back. Make sure your shoulders are squared off away from your ears. Concentrate on not moving the main part of the body as you slowly raise both feet up directly above the spine, as in **FIG. 10-2e.** Be careful that you do not create an arched feeling in your spine. If you do, tighten your buttocks and tip your pelvis. Hold this posture as long as it is comfortable. To come down, reverse the same pattern you used when going up. Rest in the fetal position for a few moments.

*TIPS*

**1.** You will find it helpful at first to do the Headstand in front of a wall. It will give you confidence, but do not let the wall become a crutch. You should not kick up to the wall. The only 2 times you should touch the wall is in FIG. 10-2c and 10-2d. And in 10-2d, it should be very lightly with the toes as you try to judge how far back to bring the feet.

**2.** When using the wall, make sure your hand grip is only three inches away. If the contour of your buttocks prevents your attaining the proper lean, in FIG. 10-2b, come down and inch your hands out a little further. Make sure not to come so far that you have to arch in FIG. 10-2d to touch the wall.

**3.** When you assume the completed Headstand, these are points to check: (1) Do not hold your breath, breathe normally. (2) Square off or widen your shoulder blades. (3) Relax your neck as you extend it, working your elbows onto the floor. (4) Your face and eyes should be relaxed. (6) Keep buttocks tight and constantly keep your heels high and pressed together as you work to find your alignment for perfect balance.

**4.** When you have achieved that perfect balance, practice again without touching the wall.

*BENEFITS*

Stimulates the flow of blood to the brain.

Firms and strengthens stomach muscles.

It is an excellent energizer. Again, this is one exercise that should definitely be a regular part of the daily routine *only* if you can do it correctly.

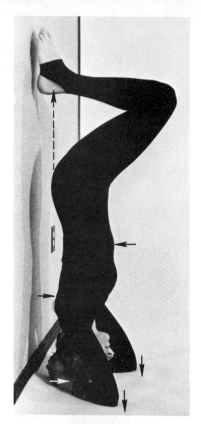

**FIG. 10-2d**

**FIG. 10-2e**

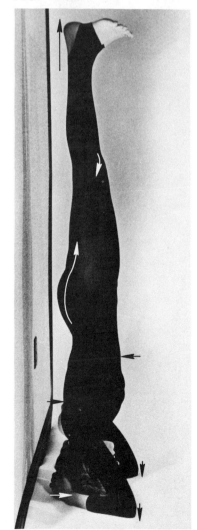

When you have mastered the Headstand well enough to do it in the middle of the room, you can go into variations which make a complete routine, bending your spine forward and backward to keep it resilient.

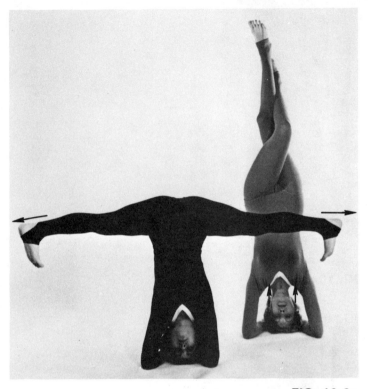
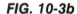

**FIG. 10-3a**

**FIG. 10-3b**

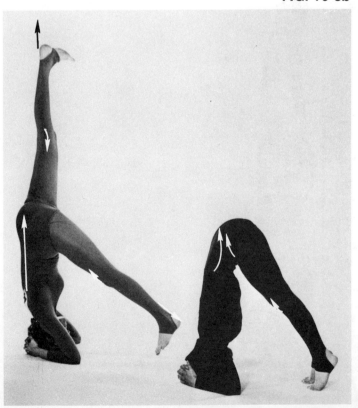

*TECHNIQUE*

1. *Leg Split:* Assume your Headstand position. Split your legs wide apart, side to side as in **FIG. 10-3a.** Then bring the legs up again. Now split the leg from front to back, going only as far as the back leg can lower, and keeping the front leg in balance with it. Make sure you do not have an arch in your back.

2. *Leg Twist:* When you can move your legs with ease, combine the motion by splitting them wide apart, rotating them from the hip in a circle, then wrapping them around each other as in **FIG. 10-3a.** Unwind and wrap in the opposite direction.

3. *Single Leg Lowering:* From the Headstand position, exhale as you lower the right leg from the waist, but do not turn your hip while you lower the left foot to the floor, as in **FIG. 10-3b.** If you must tilt the left leg in order to touch the floor, you have gone too far. Lower the right leg only to the point where you can maintain both the proper balance of your body and the vertical placement of the left leg, which is lifting high to give you balance. Inhale as you raise the right leg and repeat on the other side. In time you will be able to touch the floor.

4. *Dougle Leg Lowering:* You should attempt this only if you can master the Single Leg Lowering to the floor. Now, exhale from the Headstand position as you lower both legs together to the floor, as in **FIG. 10-3b.** In the beginning it helps to lean back very slightly as you lower, but the work is done from the hips and abdomen. Go down only as far as you can maintain control, then inhale as you go back up. If you make it down to the floor, do not rest there; barely touch and go right back up. Keep both legs straight with kneecaps raised and heels extended throughout this posture.

5. *Bent Knee:* In the Headstand position, open your legs hip-distance apart and bend your feet back at the knee. Exhale as you tighten your buttocks; lower your legs as in *FIG. 10-3c* (left). Inhale while tipping your pelvis, come up and resume your Classic Headstand.

6. *Sole Press:* From your Headstand position keeping the spine straight, exhale, press the soles of the feet together and bend the knees outward. Keep the feet directly over the crotch and lower the heels toward the crotch, as in *FIG. 10-3c* (right). (Beware that you do not arch your back but elongate.) Inhaling, bring feet back up.

7. *Bow and Arrow:* From your Headstand position arch the left leg back and place the sole of the right foot against the left knee, as in *FIG. 10-3d.* Apply a little pressure with the right foot for leverage. Keep an elongation within the spine; do not just arch the back. Come back up to a straight Headstand before repeating on the other side.

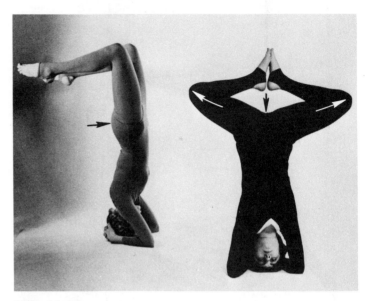

**FIG. 10-3c**

*TIPS*

1. Throughout these variations be careful not to slouch in maintaining your Headstand. Keep your shoulders and ears lifted from the floor.

2. Do not let the weight of your body come onto your neck. Keep your wrist and elbows firm on the floor, tighten your buttocks, and press ankles together as you elongate on each exhalation.

3. Maintain and lift within the spine as you execute these variations. Do not sacrifice the lift for the leg positions.

*BENEFITS*

Keeps the spine supple.
You gain more balance.
Aids in coordination.

**FIG. 10-3d**

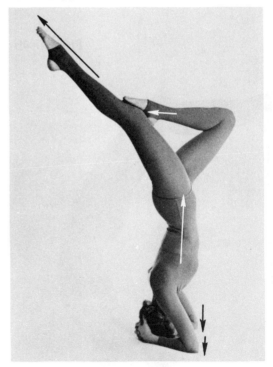

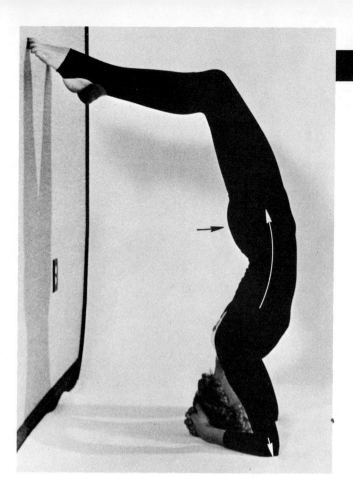

FIG. 10-4a

### TECHNIQUE

1. Do not attempt the Scorpion unless you have mastered the Headstand in the middle of the room. Kneel down in front of a wall. Bring your finger tips up against the wall. Place your right hand at your left elbow and bring the left hand down to clasp the right hand. In general, this guide works for most of my students, but it can be adjusted to suit you, depending on the arch in your body.

2. Proceed now to do a regular Headstand. Once you are up and balanced, bend your legs until your toes touch the wall, as in *FIG. 10-4a.* Make sure you keep the support and weight on your elbows.

3. Unclasp the hands and place them on the floor. With elbows and flat palms, jointly apply pressure onto the floor, and push against the wall with your toes. Thus, you attain leverage to lift the shoulders and raise your head up from the floor, as in *FIG. 10-4b.*

FIG. 10-4b

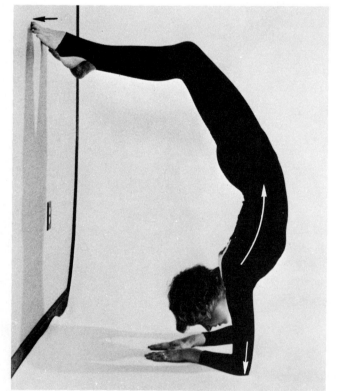

4. Ease the pressure that you have been applying on the wall as you shift the weight and balance onto the elbows, forearms, wrists and palms. Your head should be in the center of your forearms, not over your hands (see *FIG. 10-4c*). If you concentrate on this, you will find that the body automatically acquires an inner balance which will enable you to hold this posture without touching the wall (see *FIG. 10-4d*). Hold for the count of 5. Bend forward at the waist and drop the feet gently to the floor. Rest in the fetal position.

*TIPS*

1. Before your toes leave the wall, make sure you feel the supportive strength and contraction in your squared off shoulders, arms, elbows and palms. Remember, pull your head back away from over your hands.

2. If you find yourself losing your balance, spring away from the wall and bring your feet down to the floor instead of collapsing, or you might fall on your face.

3. I would not encourage those of you who have a sway back to do the Scorpion too often. When you do assume this posture, it is not the arch that gives you balance but the lift up throughout the body.

*BENEFITS*

Tones and gives a concave stretch to the spine.
Develops strength in the arms, shoulders and abdominal wall.
Expands the chest.

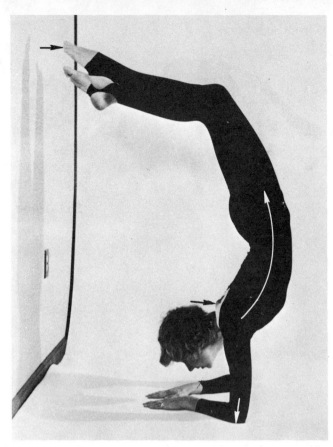

**FIG. 10-4c**

**FIG. 10-4d**

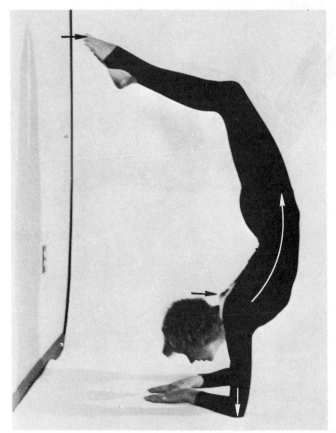

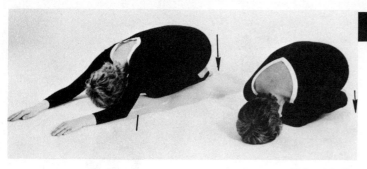

FIG. 10-5a

### Mecca Pose

*TECHNIQUE*

1. Place yourself so you are on your hands and knees. Keeping your hands in that position, inhale.
2. Sitting back on your heels, exhale as you rest head on floor in front of your knees.
3. Keeping the stretch in the arms, bend the elbows, as in *FIG. 10-5a* (left). Relax, breathing normally.

### Classic Fetal Pose

*TECHNIQUE*

1. Inhale, kneel, and sit back on your heels. Exhale, rest your head on the floor in front of your knees.
2. Bring both hands back toward the toes and rest hands on the floor, with elbows bent, as in *FIG. 10-5a* (right). Relax in this position, breathing normally.

### Shoulder Relaxer

*TECHNIQUE*

1. Assume the Fetal Position with your forehead right against your knees. Inhale, clasping your hands behind.
2. Shrug your shoulders back, making a tight shoulder blade squeeze. Exhale as you raise the arms up over the head with hands still clasped and elbows straight. As you stretch the straight arms up higher, proceed to raise the buttocks up from the floor, as in *FIG. 10-5b.* Make sure you keep your shoulders raised from the floor.
3. To get more of a stretch from this position when you are up, as in *FIG. 10-5b,* walk the knees closer to the forehead. Stay to the count of 3–5 breaths as you continue to stretch into the move. Then relax in the Classic Fetal Position.

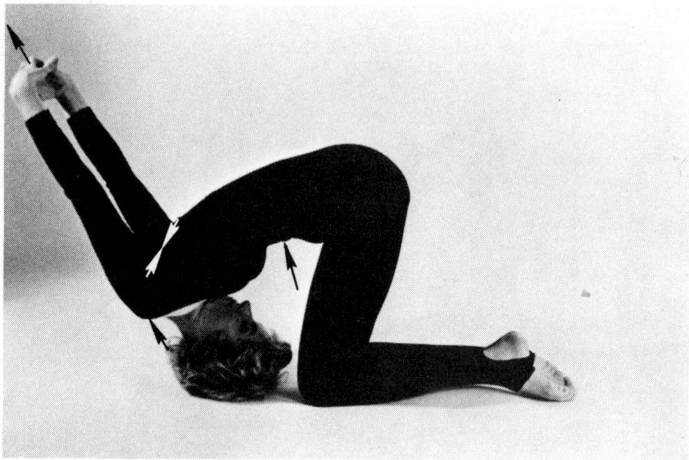

FIG. 10-5b

## Neck Relaxer

### TECHNIQUE

From the Classic Fetal Position, inhale; then exhale as you raise your buttocks up, letting your arms relax and slide with you as you move forward. Inhale, keep the head in the forward position, but as you exhale and lift from the neck and shoulders, feel the forward movement in the scalp. You are elongating the neck as in *FIG. 10-5c.* Keep stretching in this position for 3–4 breaths.

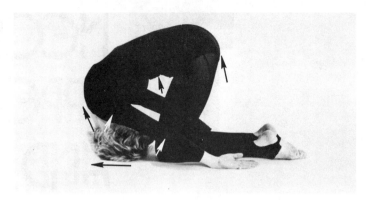

**FIG. 10-5c**

## Dolphin Pose

### TECHNIQUE

1. Assume the Shoulder Relaxer Pose without walking the feet in. Your feet can either be together or hip-distance apart.
2. Curl your toes under, lift shoulders away from the floor. Inhale, then exhaling, straighten out your legs, as in *FIG. 10-5d.* Do not roll back on the head. Stay on top and lift neck up. Take 3 breaths and slowly come down.

### TIPS

1. In the Mecca Pose and Classic Pose, you may find it too difficult to sit back on your heels, so place a pillow under your forehead.
2. Breathe naturally and keep your facial muscles relaxed.
3. Concentrate on working the shoulders or neck as the exercise indicates.

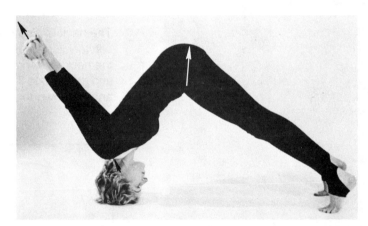

**FIG. 10-5d**

### BENEFITS

Relaxes the lower back.
Eases neck and shoulder tension.
Regulates the flow of blood.

# 11 NECK, UPPER BACK AND CHEST

The neck is also part of the spine, since the first seven vertebrae (called the cervical vertebrae) form the neck. The group of muscles you feel while doing the neck stretches are the sternomastoids, which come from behind the ears and go down to the sternum, and the trapezius, which originate behind the ear and go down the shoulders, as in *DIAGRAM 1.*

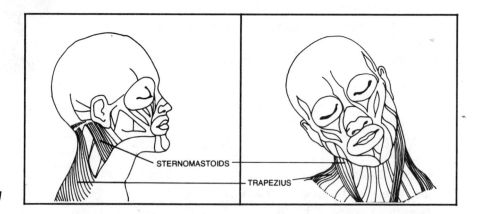

*Diagram 1*

STERNOMASTOIDS

TRAPEZIUS

If the carriage and balance of the neck is too far forward or backward, the balance of the entire body can be affected. Tightening in any one area of the spine or chest may produce misalignment in the entire body, especially in the vertebral column.

When you are lying down doing floor exercises, be very careful not to raise the chin toward the ceiling. Do not arch the neck. Instead, use the following correct position: elongate the back of the neck and tuck in the chin. Then relax the chin, but keep the neck elongated.

Correct placement of the neck is vital to the whole body. The thoracic extensor straightens the thoracic portion of the spine so that the entire spine improves its alignment.

Proper neck alignment with the spine makes good breathing habits easier. To avoid stiffness and tension, the correct position of the head and neck should rate particular attention throughout all the exercises.

With the neck in proper position, the correct placement of the squeezed shoulder blades is assured. Lifting the complete cervical spine from the floor will in turn facilitate the extension of the sternum (**DIAGRAM 2**) and enable the spine to arch properly for the postures that follow in this book.

CERVICAL SPINE OFF FLOOR

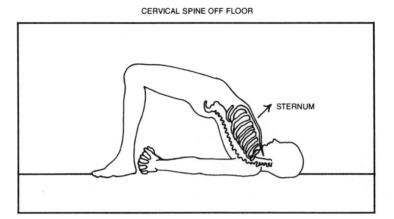

STERNUM

**Diagram 2**

85

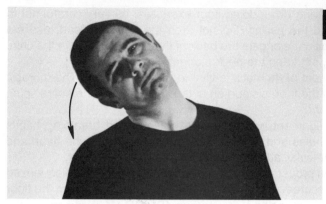

FIG. 11-1a

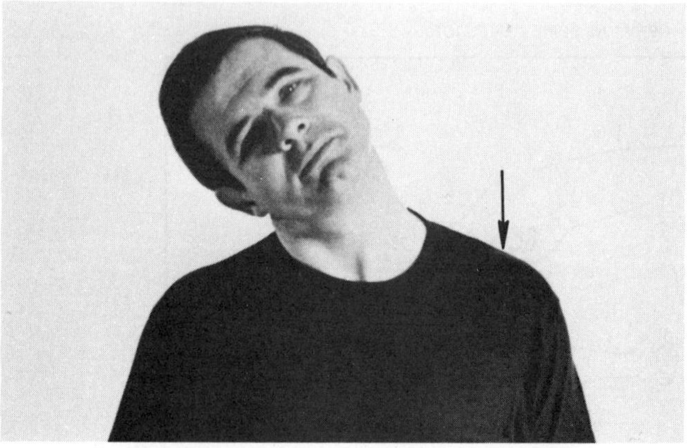

### TECHNIQUE

1. Sit on the floor in a cross-legged position, or sit in a chair, but do not lean back on the chair. It is very important to have your spine straight.
2. Inhale, extending sternum as you elongate the neck. Exhale as you tilt the head to the right, lowering your ear toward the shoulder *(FIG.11-1a)*. Keep the shoulder relaxed and do not raise it.
3. Inhale, sit taller, maintaining the tilt. Exhale as you lower the left shoulder, feeling the muscles tautly pulled *(FIG. 11-1b)*. This is the sternomastoid muscle that runs from the back of the ear down to the shoulder. I want you to feel this strong pull in the neck.
4. Inhaling, raise the head to the upright position. Repeat the same to the left side. Keep looking straight ahead.
5. Inhale, elongating the neck. Exhale as you project the chin forward and continue downward to the chest *(FIG. 11-1c)*. Keep the shoulders relaxed.
6. Inhale, extending sternum, stretch forward from the chin. Exhale as you slowly continue projecting chin forward and upward. Extend the chin toward the ceiling *(FIG. 11-1d)*. Do not just drop the head back. Keep shoulders and back of the neck relaxed. Do not slouch, keep a straight back.
7. Inhaling, lead with the chin, bringing it up and around in front. Then return to the balanced position.
8. Repeat the complete set of positions 4 times.

### TIPS

1. The reason I emphasize the strong stretch in the sternomastoid muscle is that this relieves pressure and stimulates the circulation of blood to the brain.
2. One of the causes of headaches is tension build-up, which restricts the blood flow in the head.
3. Keep in mind the rhythm of your breath as you relax within the 4 Tilts.
4. Do not rush through the position. Take time to feel the benefits while within each position.

### BENEFITS

Beneficial for migraine headaches.
Relieves tension in the neck.
Eases a stiff neck.

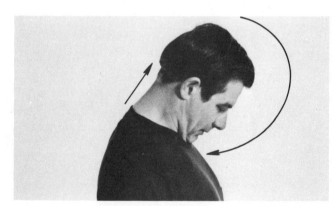

FIG. 11-1b

FIG. 11-1c

FIG. 11-1d

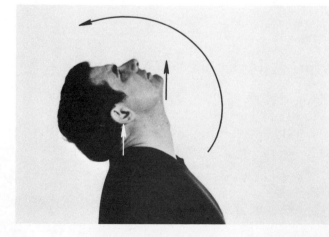

## TECHNIQUE

1. Sit on the floor with crossed legs or in a chair. It does not matter which position you assume, but you must have a straight back.

2. Inhale, and elongate the neck. Exhale as you project the chin forward, and continue downward to the chest, tucking in the chin and stretching the back of the neck *(FIG. 11-2a)*. Keep shoulder down!

3. Inhale, extending sternum; stretch forward from the chin. Continue projecting the chin to the ceiling. Exhale with a lift in the neck, let the head drop back as far as possible, keeping the mouth closed *(FIG. 11-2b)*. Do not hunch the shoulders. Keep them down and back.

4. Keeping the lift in the neck, open the mouth. This will make the head drop further back *(FIG. 11-2c)*. Keep shoulders down.

5. Keeping the head in the far back position, close your mouth and then extend your lower jaw forward and up *(FIG. 11-2d)*. This will give a good stretch to your neck and chin.

6. With your mouth closed, inhale as you elongate your neck.

7. Exhale as you extend the chin up, extend forward, around, and down. This will bring the chin back down *(FIG. 11-2a)*.

## TIPS

1. If you have difficulty dropping the head back as in Step 3, FIG. 11-2b, you may lean your body back a bit.

2. It is most important to keep a straight back throughout this whole stretch.

3. Do not just drop your head back. First, lift the neck and stretch the shoulders down.

## BENEFITS

Smooths the skin of the neck and chest.
Helps alleviate double chin.
Relieves tension in the neck.

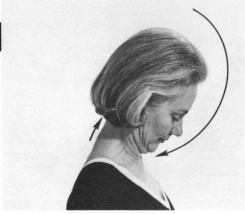

**FIG. 11-2a**

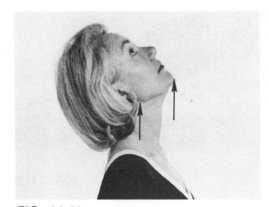

**FIG. 11-2b**

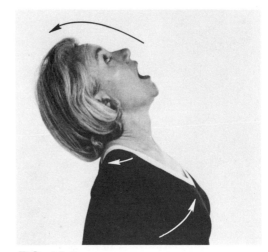

**FIG. 11-2c**

**FIG. 11-2d**

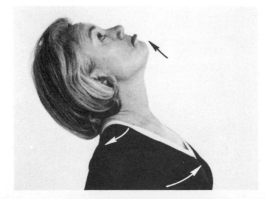

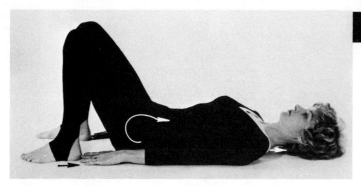

**FIG. 11-3a**

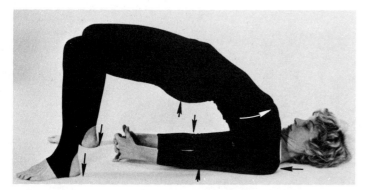

**FIG. 11-3b**

### TECHNIQUE

1. Lie down, bend your knees with feet hip-distance apart so that the heels come to the tips of your fingers. Adjust your head so your neck is elongated, as in **FIG. 11-3a.**

2. Inhaling, tip your pelvis as you press onto the floor with the balls of the feet and heels. Exhaling, roll your buttocks up, then slowly one vertebra at a time, continuing to roll up the spinal column while pressing your shoulders on the floor, as in **FIG. 11-3b.**

3. Now with straight arms on the floor, clasp your hands beneath you and squeeze your shoulder blades together while walking your shoulders in together and away from your neck. Your cervical spine should be lifted completely from the floor.

4. While in this arched position, inhale, extending the sternum. Exhale while you tighten the buttocks, lifting yourself higher. See **FIG. 11-3b.** Work to lift your hips up high toward the ceiling, not into the neck. You also extend the sternum toward the chin, not chin to sternum, which will create tension in the throat.

5. Do this for 3 rounds of breathing as you accomplish a better lift. To come down, raise your arms and fingers to the ceiling. Exhale as you tip your pelvis and slowly roll down, letting your shoulder blades touch down first, then your waist, and lastly, your buttocks. Relax.

6. For more of a stretch, slide your feet and ankles together, still keeping heels at finger-tip alignment. Inhale and apply the same technique as in Steps 2–5, but when you arrive at your ultimate height without sagging, squeeze your knees together, as in **FIG. 11-3c.**

7. While in **FIG. 11-3c,** take 3 breaths with your hands unclasped, but keep elbows in the same position.

8. Do not continue unless you have a good lift, as in **FIG. 11-3c,** not just an arch, to attain the techniques of Steps 9–10.

9. Inhaling, extend the sternum. Exhaling, tighten and lift the buttocks. Inhale as you raise your left leg, but only to the point where the knees and thighs remain together at a 45° angle. Exhale as you now bring the left leg completely up, lifting the buttocks at the same time. Inhale while reaching your left leg and heel toward the ceiling, making sure the leg is perpendicular to the floor, as in **FIG. 11-3d.**

10. Keeping your leg up, raise both arms toward the ceiling, releasing the squeeze in the shoulder blades. Exhale as you slowly roll one vertebra at a time to the floor. Then bend at the knee to return the left foot to meet the right foot.

11. Repeat the same with the right leg.

12. To come down, repeat as in Step 5.

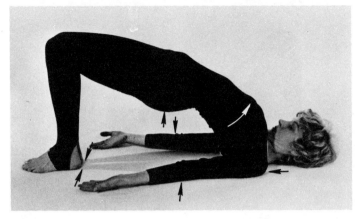

FIG. 11-3c

### TIPS

1. Throughout this posture, we concentrate first on the extension of the sternum, then on tightening and lifting the buttocks. If this is done correctly, you will not feel tension in the lower back but get the straight elongation throughout the whole spine.

2. In all variations it is very important to have your feet straight, not at an angle, and your heels directly below your knees. From heels to finger tips is only an average gauge. You may need to vary the distance.

3. Make sure you do not open your knees out to the side in any variation, whether it be feet apart or feet together, when you are up in the raised position. The tibia or shin bone must be perpendicular to the floor.

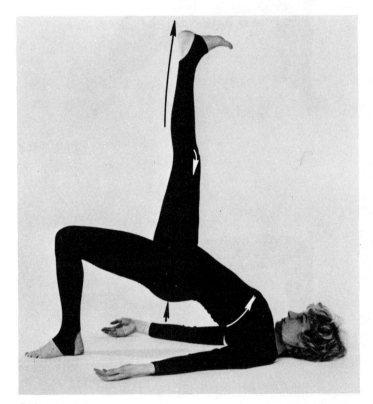

FIG. 11-3d

### BENEFITS

Limbers up the spine
Works off fatty deposits and firms the legs, thighs, hips, and abdomen.
Loosens neck and shoulder region.

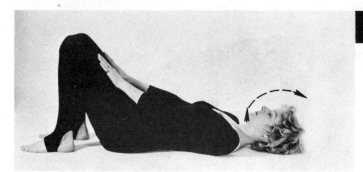

**FIG. 11-4a**

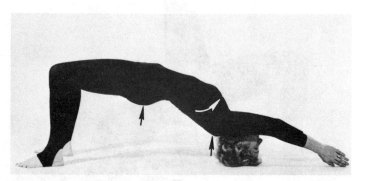

top of head

**FIG. 11-4b**

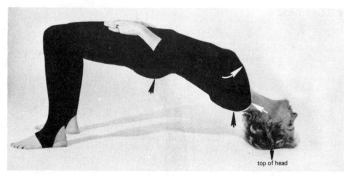

**FIG. 11-4c**

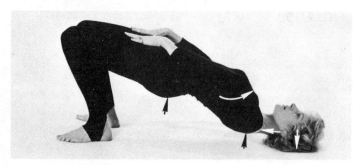

**FIG. 11-4d**

## TECHNIQUE

1. Lie down with hands on thighs and bring your feet directly under your knees, hip-distance apart, as in **FIG. 11-4a.** Inhaling, raise your sternum and chin while tucking head under.

2. Exhale as you raise your spine and buttocks, stretching the neck up and pulling your shoulders away from your ears, as in **FIG. 11-4b.** You are applying a direct lift with your sternum and hips toward the ceiling while you tighten your buttocks, so as not to crest a bend in the neck but work to elongate the neck.

3. Inhaling again, lift shoulders, and extend sternum. Then exhale as you continue to tighten the buttocks and reach up further, creating a lift throughout the whole body.

4. Inhale once again applying all of the above techniques. Exhale as you bring the hands up from the thighs and backward over your head to the floor, as in **FIG. 11-4c.** Inhale and lift shoulders from the floor. Exhaling, lift into your perfect Bridge.

5. To come out, return hands to thighs, press the head onto the floor and slowly roll down along the back of the head, applying pressure with head to floor as you keep the shoulders raised, as in **FIG. 11-4d.** Feel the release in the neck. Now, proceed to lower the shoulders and continue down as in Shoulder Bridge.

## TIPS

1. This is a Head Bridge since the balance comes from the head, not in the neck. You are continually working shoulders away from the ears and floor to free the neck.

2. Make sure you do not roll too far back on the head. You balance slightly to the back of the top of the head.

## BENEFITS

Strengthens neck and spine.
Stimulates the scalp.
Tones thighs.

### TECHNIQUE

1. Lie down, bending your knees so the feet come directly under your knees and hip-distance apart. Lift up and clasp your hands, elbows straight with little fingers on the floor, elongating the back of the neck and squeezing the shoulder blades together and away from the neck, lifting the cervical spine off the floor.

2. Inhale, extending the sternum. Exhale as you raise the spine further. Keeping the elbows in close, place your wrists above your waist, cupping your lower back with your hands, as in **FIG. 11-5a.**

3. Inhale, extend the sternum, and bring your right knee toward the ceiling, raising to the toes of your left foot.

4. Exhale as you complete the cycles by swinging the right toes over head to the floor. The left leg follows behind, as in **FIG. 11-5c.** Continue to lower the left foot to bring the legs together. Now you are in the Plough Pose.

5. Inhale, elongate, raise your right knee toward the ceiling as you tighten the buttocks and extend the hip forward, as in **FIG. 11-5d.** Now slowly lower the right foot to the floor, keeping the hips high. Let the left leg follow behind, as in **FIG. 11-5b.**

6. Next, leading with the right leg, do Steps 2–5 for 3 more full cycles. When completed, slowly lower feet to the floor, as in **FIG. 11-5a.**

7. Now, raise and reach fingers toward the ceiling, slowly roll out of it as you tip your pelvis, letting your shoulder blades touch first, then waist and lastly your buttocks.

### TIPS

1. To lift the right leg, spring up gently with the left toes, as in FIG. 5b, continuing with a very light rhythmic swing as you *lightly* touch the floor.

2. It is important to maintain the lift, so apply pressure onto the ribs with your hands and wrists, keeping the elbows directly under the hands.

3. As in FIG. 11-5d, Step 5, concentrate on extending the hips high as well as forward while rotating down.

### BENEFITS

Makes spine healthy and flexible.
Strengthens wrists and arms.
Develops coordination.

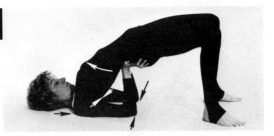

**FIG. 11-5a**

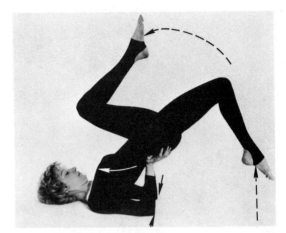

**FIG. 11-5b**

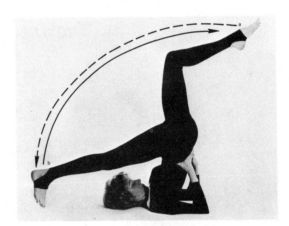

**FIG. 11-5c**

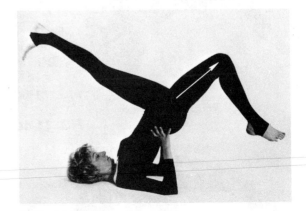

**FIG. 11-5d**

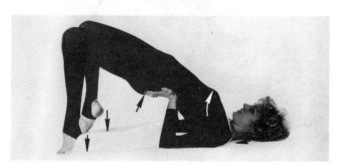

FIG. 11-6a

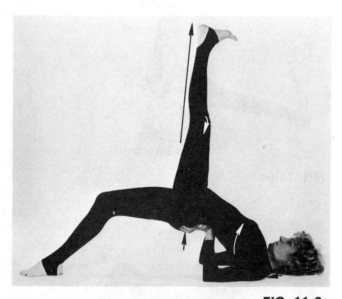

FIG. 11-6b

FIG. 11-6c

FIG. 11-6d

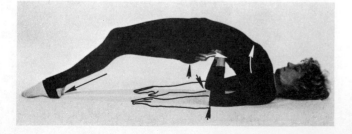

### TECHNIQUE

1. Assume the Plough Pose with hands clasped behind you. Elongate the back of the neck and squeeze the shoulder blades together and away from the neck, lifting the cervical spine off the floor. With elbows as close as possible, place your wrists just onto your waist, and cup the buttocks with your hands.

2. Inhale, extending sternum. Exhale as you tighten buttocks and rotate the hips, bringing legs up, as in **FIG. 11-6a.**

3. Inhale, increasing your arch. Exhale as you bend the knees, keeping your buttocks tight and hips forward while slowly and *lightly* lowering your legs to the floor, as in **FIG. 11-6b.**

4. Now with your ankles and knees together, slide your feet down to where the legs are as straight as you can make them, with toes and heels still on the floor.

5. Inhale, extending the sternum and lift. Exhale as you raise your left heel toward the ceiling, as in **FIG. 11-6c.**

6. Inhale, reaching the heel up further as if to lengthen the leg. Exhale, extending the heel as you lower the leg to the floor. Repeat with the right leg.

7. With both legs touching at the knees and ankles, inhale. Maintain your lift, and exhale as you work the hand further up the back, as in **FIG. 11-6d.** Take 3 more breaths in this position, concentrating on keeping the lift in your spine.

8. On your last exhalation, lower your arms to the floor and slide your feet down so you rest on the floor. Reward yourself with some nice deep relaxing breaths. You deserve it.

### TIPS

1. Your shoulder, not spine, should be pressing onto the floor at all times. This helps your balance.

2. To lessen the pressure on the wrists and hands, concentrate on extending the sternum, elongating the spine, and keeping heels firmly on the floor.

### BENEFITS

Builds a flexible spine which, in turn, yields a healthy nervous system.
If done correctly, removes strain in the neck.
Develops balance.

# 12 FORWARD FLEXIBILITY OF THE LOWER SPINE

At first you may find the Plough posture difficult to execute, especially if you have a stiff spine and shortened back muscles. Forcing yourself, as in **DIAGRAM 1,** will only strain the spine and may hurt your neck. You are also apt to experience the sensation of shock or suffocation as a result of pressure caused by incorrect placement of the neck.

To feel and understand the correct approach, rest your leg on a chair, as in **DIAGRAM 2.** Clasp the palms together, creating a blade squeeze strong enough to lift the cervical (neck) vertebrae completely from the floor. Keeping the lift, place the heel of your index finger just below the shoulder blades. Concave the spine as you rotate the hip to bring the perineum (crotch) toward the ceiling, extending the ischium bones as high as you can. This stretch of the spine will relieve pressure on the lungs, neck, and abdomen. The movements

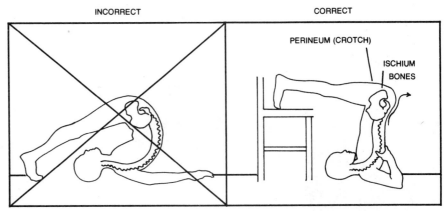

INCORRECT · CORRECT

PERINEUM (CROTCH)

ISCHIUM BONES

*Diagram 1* · *Diagram 2*

of the Plough and the breathing rhythm (inhale, elongate; exhale, concave) should occur smoothly and simultaneously for as long as you are comfortable in this posture. The tendency at first is to move in an uneven or jerky fashion, but this is usually overcome when the student slowly and deliberately applies the breathing rhythm while analyzing each move. Inhale and lift; pause in the position; exhale and move. Smoothness and continuity will come with practice.

Work on the Plough until you acquire the ability to stretch and relax all the inter-vertebral muscles in the dorsal region. You will notice that improved spinal pliability and suppleness add ease and grace to your carriage.

Of course, the ease or difficulty of the action will depend on the individual's weight or body type. People whose spines are bony need extra protection against bruising during the Rock and Roll. I recommend doubling the thickness of the mat or carpet for these folks. Make sure that the double protection extends for the length of the entire body and not just in the particular area that is sensitive, for in order to keep aligned, the head, neck, and spine must be level. The knees should be straight during these postures for maximum benefits.

By practicing these postures, movements will be increased in a spine stiffened from nervous tension, calcium deposits, or arthritis. The value of the Plough and its related postures lies in opening the intervertebral spaces, allowing the back muscles and spine to stretch.

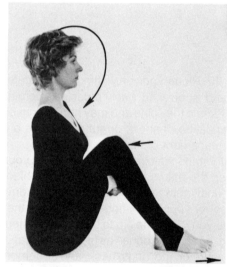

FIG. 12-1a
FIG. 12-1b

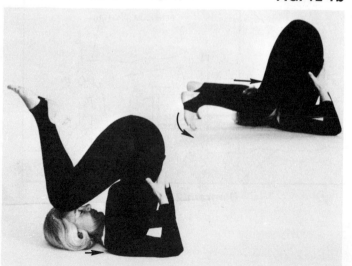

## ROCK AND ROLL

### TECHNIQUE

1. Sit up and bend knees to chest, with hands under the knees, as in **FIG. 12-1a.**

2. Tuck your head in and keep it tucked in as you push with your feet and swing, letting yourself go to get the momentum to rock back and forth. Do this about 5 times.

3. Now, hold the position where you are on your shoulders with your knees on your forehead. Take your hands and hold your back, as in **FIG. 12-1b** (left). Make sure you are pressing the shoulders onto the floor, *not* your spine.

4. Spread your knees apart and drop them to the shoulders. You must keep your thighs against your chest and your back into your hands. Don't roll forward. If you are doing this correctly, there will not be any strain in the neck.

5. Keeping the thighs against the chest, exhale rolling slightly forward. Do not let the thighs move, but lower the legs enough to allow your toes to touch the floor, with knees remaining by shoulders and feet at right angle, as in **FIG. 12-1b** (right). Remember, face and neck are relaxed.

6. Without moving toes from this exact spot, you straighten your legs by letting the hips lean onto your hands, as in *FIG. 12-1c.* If your legs will not straighten completely, that is all right. They will in time. The important point is that there be no tension in the neck.

7. To come out, bend your knee back to your forehead, placing the hands behind your knees, as in *FIG. 12-1d.* As you fold the legs, bring the heel toward your buttocks and roll up, as in *FIG. 12-1a.*

8. When you can be in the *FIG. 12-1c* position with no tension in your neck or shoulders while your toes are on the floor, you may continue on to rock back and forth, maintaining a smooth momentum. If you find tension, use the chair technique shown in *DIAGRAM 2.*

9. So let us sit up once again. Bring knees to chest, exhale as you tuck your head down.

10. Inhale as you roll back on your shoulders, hands under your knees, as in *FIG. 12-1d.*

11. Exhale as you straighten out the legs, keeping hands behind the knees, with toes on the floor, as in *FIG. 12-1c.*

12. Now bend knees back to your forehead. Inhale as you fold the legs up and get momentum to roll up. Repeat Steps 9–12 five more times until you have really loosened your spine.

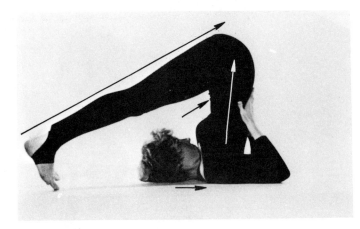

**FIG. 12-1c**

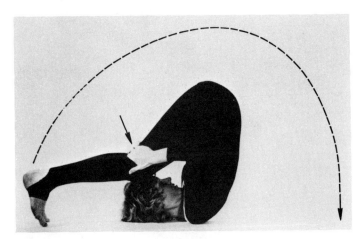

**FIG. 12-1d**

### TIPS

1. If you have trouble touching the floor with your toes, rest your feet against a wall as you rock back. As you loosen up, you can walk your toes down the wall. This is explained in my first book under "Walking Down the Wall."

2. Make sure that you apply a good exhalation when you are trying to reach the floor with your toes. It can make a big difference.

3. Make this fun. Just let yourself roll back and forth.

### BENEFITS

Strengthens and coordinates the whole body while massaging the neck and spine.
Stimulates the thyroid gland.
Relieves tension in head and neck.
Great energizer.

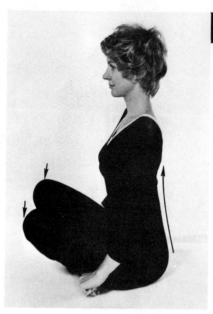

FIG. 12-2a

*TECHNIQUE*

1. Do not try this exercise until you can easily do the Rock and Roll. Sit on the floor tailor fashion with your hands holding your toes, as in *FIG. 12-2a.* Keep holding the toes throughout this entire posture.
2. Exhale, tummy in, inhale as you elongate. Leading with the sternum, exhale as you lower the head to the floor in front of you, at the same time keeping the buttocks on the floor, as in *FIG. 12-2b.*

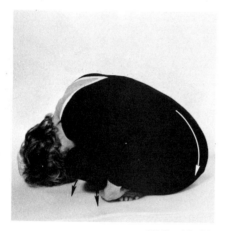

FIG. 12-2b

3. Inhale as you roll back. Do not let go of your feet. Exhale as you bring your toes to the floor behind your head, still grasping the toes, as in **FIG. 12-2c.**

4. Work to straighten the back, reaching the perineum toward the ceiling. Concentrate on breathing slowly as you work to straighten the legs, as in **FIG. 12-2d.**

5. To lower the body, bend the knees to the chest. Inhale as you let your buttocks drop down onto the floor. Still grasping the toes, pull the feet against the back of the thighs and swing the knees forward and down. This will bring you up to a sitting position, as in **FIG. 12-2a.** Exhale as you rest your forehead on the floor in front of you. Repeat this posture 3 more times. Then reverse your legs and repeat.

6. To get more stretch out of this exercise when you are in **FIG. 12-2d,** inhale, elongating the back and raising hips. Exhaling, feel the stretch down the legs as you extend your heels away and pull your toes in toward your head. (Note my hand grip in **FIG. 12-2d**).

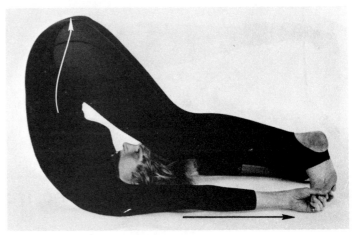

**FIG. 12-2c**

## TIPS

1. To accomplish FIG. 12-2b, pull your feet out to the sides as you lower knees toward the floor. This will bring the head further down.
2. You should work toward building up a coordinated rhythmic motion as you rock back and forth.
3. Do not cross your arms.

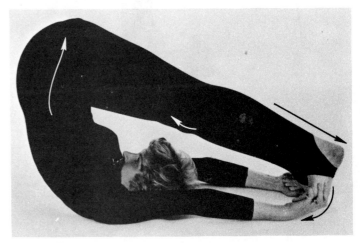

**FIG. 12-2d**

## BENEFITS

An excellent exercise to massage the entire spine from neck to the lower tip.
Slims and firms thighs and hips.
Improves circulation.

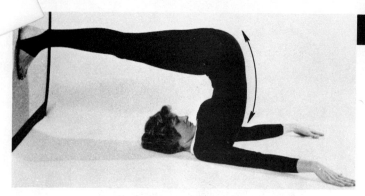

**FIG. 12-3a**

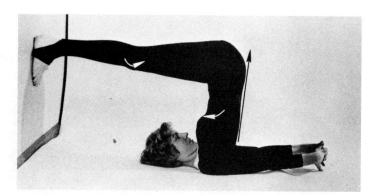

**FIG. 12-3b**

*TECHNIQUE*

1. Sit with your back to the wall, approximately 4–5 feet away.
2. Rock back and straighten your legs so your toes and heels are flat against the wall and your legs are parallel to the floor, as in *FIG. 12-3a.* You are too far from the wall if this is uncomfortable in the throat or neck.
3. In this position, inhale, clasping your hands behind you on the floor. Straighten arms (elbows in), squeeze shoulder blades together, and shrug shoulders down away from your ears. Exhale as you lift up your hips to elongate and straighten your back, making a right angle with the legs, as in *FIG. 12-3b.* Your cervical spine should be recessed and completely off the floor.
4. Place your hands as high as possible toward the shoulders. Move the skin of neck and shoulder area out of the way in the direction of the waist, so the hands ultimately grip a taut back. Keep elbows in as close to each other as possible.

5. Walk the toes up the wall about one foot. Pushing heels away from the wall with the toes, raise your kneecaps toward the thighs, while concaving the spine as you work your hands further onto the back and just under the shoulder blades, as in *FIG. 12-3c.*

6. In this position, inhale extending the sternum while lifting and elongating the spine. Exhaling, further concave the back as you lift up, extending your perineum (crotch) toward the ceiling. Notice the relief in your neck and breathing.

7. Repeat Step 6 three times with the suggested breathing rhythm. When balance is achieved, you will find your spine recessed and your toes off the wall entirely, as in *FIG. 12-3d* (left).

8. To come down, keep kneecaps raised and heels extended as you lower. Exhaling slowly, lower your legs to the floor without moving your back or changing the placement of your hips.

9. When toes reach the floor, place your hands on the back of your leg at the ankles. Wing out your elbows, raise your kneecaps, extend your heel, working to bring your straight legs close to the face, as in *FIG. 12-3d* (right). Continue slowly rolling down on the spine, one vertebra at a time.

10. When your buttocks reach the floor, let go and place your hands at your sides, using them as brakes while you tip your pelvis, pressing the small of the back on the floor as you lower the legs down. Only lower the legs as far as you can while still maintaining the back on the floor. Then bend legs, placing feet on the floor.

11. This was a hard and detailed exercise. You deserve to relax and take some nice deep Rib Cage Breaths.

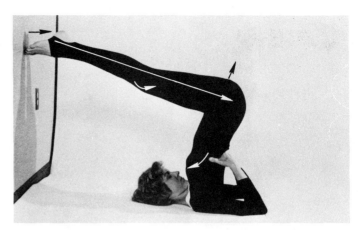

**FIG. 12-3c**

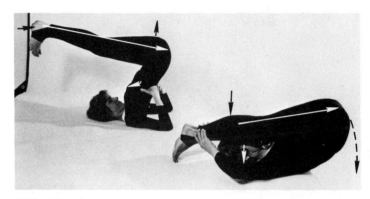

**FIG. 12-3d**

## TIPS

1. When you can master Steps 1–7 correctly, attempt this whole procedure without the wall. Make sure your cervical spine is off the floor throughout.

2. I know you will want to slouch in this posture, but it puts a great deal of pressure on your neck and chest. Keep elongating, reaching high with your ischium bone and perineum as you work this pose. Keep in mind *you* can control your body. Do not let *it* control you.

## BENEFITS

An excellent massage for the entire spinal column.
Strengthens and stretches the hamstrings.
Relieves stiff shoulders and arthritis of the back.

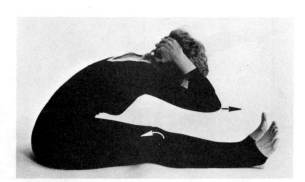

FIG. 12-4a

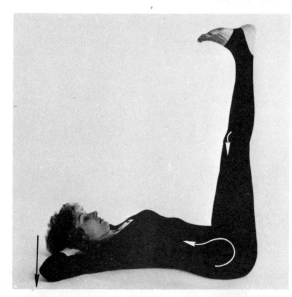

FIG. 12-4b

## TECHNIQUE

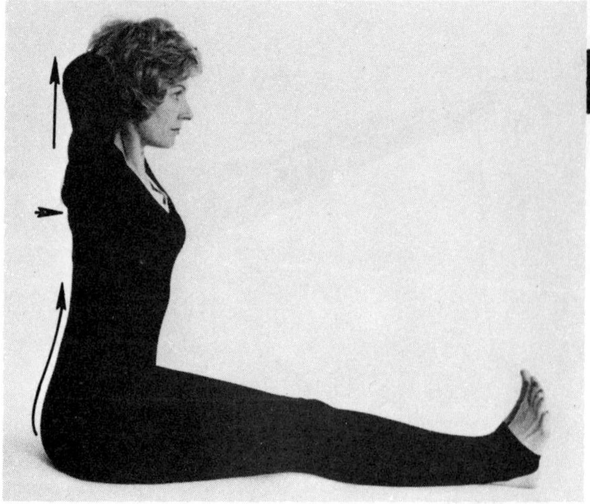

1. Lie down with back flat on the floor. Inhale as you interlace the fingers at the back of the head.
2. Exhaling, tip your pelvis and raise your shoulders as you proceed to roll the spine back up.
3. Inhale into a nice high, straight sitting position, as in *FIG. 12-4a,* with elbows high.
4. Exhaling, reach out in front while lowering your elbows, reaching as far down the legs as possible, as in *FIG. 12-4b.*
5. Inhaling, roll the spine back up with elbows high to the sitting position, as in *FIG. 12-4a.* Exhaling, slowly roll the spine down to the floor.
6. Inhale, tip pelvis. Exhale as you raise the legs up, as in *FIG. 12-4c.* Applying the Tummy-In action, further tip the pelvis to roll the lower back from the floor and exhale into the Plough Pose, as in *FIG. 12-4d.*
7. Take a small breath and proceed to exhale as you lower the spine, vertebra by vertebra, to the floor, as in *FIG. 12-4c.*
8. Keeping your head down, continue slowly to lower the legs to the floor by tipping your pelvis and keeping your back down onto the floor.
9. Repeat these 8 Steps for 5–10 times. Do not rush. Stretch in a deliberate fashion in each position.

## TIPS

1. If this hand position is too difficult, place hands out in front of you with your thumbs interlocked, or just let your hands slide to cup your ears instead of the back of your head.
2. In FIG. 12-4d move the hands to the top of the head so that the head will be flat on the floor.

## BENEFITS

Complete massage of the spine and neck.
Slims the waist, hips and thighs.
Very good for circulation.

FIG. 12-4c

FIG. 12-4d

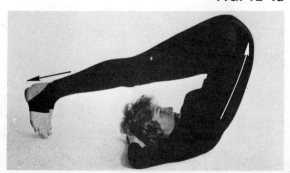

### TECHNIQUE

1. Sit on the floor, knees bent with hands under them, as in **FIG. 12-5a.**

2. Inhale as you push with feet and roll back until your knees are on your forehead. Exhale as you separate the knees, bringing them to rest by the ears and shoulders, as in **FIG. 12-5b.** Exhaling further, keeping a lift within the spine, tilt the body toward your chin and lower the knees closer to the floor.

3. Inhaling, grasp the instep of the right foot with both hands. Pull the foot with your hands and push the knee into the shoulder, keeping the knee on the floor. Exhale as you raise the left leg, as in **FIG. 12-5c.** Inhaling, raise up the left heel toward the ceiling, keeping the leg as straight as possible. Exhale as you slowly lower your left leg to the floor. Repeat the above step using the right leg.

4. Now that you are a little more limber, you are going to try to get both knees to rest flat on the floor against the shoulders. Rest both forearms on the backs of the knees, and work your fingers between the knees and the head, so that the palms are cupping both ears, as in **FIG. 12-5d.**

5. Believe it or not, this posture can be most relaxing. Hold this position, taking 3–5 normal breaths, or until you want to come out of it. Slowly roll out of this position with control.

### TIPS

1. In FIG. 12-5c, you acquire the balance for raising the leg by pulling the knee toward the shoulder, winging out the elbows and pressing them onto the floor.

2. In FIG. 12-5d, note that working your arms and hands into this position helps get your knees lower and gives the balance you need.

3. Do not collapse your chest. Keep a straight lift within the spine so you can breathe easily.

### BENEFITS

Excellent for stretching the spine.
Slims and firms thighs and hips.
Massages all the internal organs.

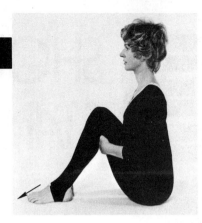

**FIG. 12-5a**

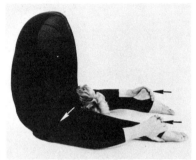

**FIG. 12-5b**

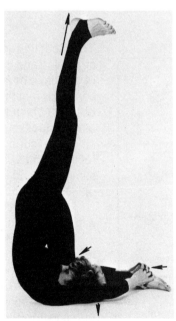

**FIG. 12-5c**

**FIG. 12-5d**

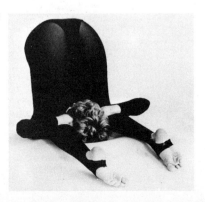

# 13 SHOULDER STAND

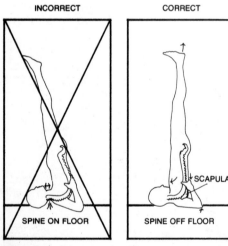

INCORRECT

CORRECT

SPINE ON FLOOR

SPINE OFF FLOOR

SCAPULA

**Diagram 1**          **Diagram 2**

The great therapeutic value of the Shoulder Stand lies in a dual mechanism of stretching and isometric contraction on three distinct muscular groups, stretch of the back muscles, contraction of the muscles in the abdominal wall, and contraction of the fore muscles of the neck. The cervical section of the spinal column (which houses a network of nerves) is lifted from the floor in a tight blade squeeze, and is freed, toned up and generally revived.

The substantial increase in the supply of blood to the brain aids in relieving the vascular spasms that are so often responsible for headaches, stimulates and improves the function of the thryoid, thymus, and parathyroid glands and contributes to the general well-being of the entire human organism.

With the contraction and relaxation of the visceral muscles comes the elimination of digestive, metabolic, urinary, and uterine ailments.

*DIAGRAM 1* shows conjested lungs, with the weight of the body being felt on the neck and head, and a lack of tone in the abdomen and legs, thus throwing the body all out of alignment.

In *DIAGRAM 2,* you see a nicely aligned Shoulder Stand. On each inhalation, bring the *sternum to the chin* and *not* the chin to the sternum. Bringing the chin to the sternum will tend to create tension and a collapsed lung position. Bringing the sternum to the chin will help to expand the chest and bring the body into the correct balanced position on the shoulders, thus its name—not a neck lean.

### TECHNIQUE

1. Back a chair against a wall so chair will not slip. Lie on the floor, place lower legs on the chair seat, with your buttocks and thighs in line with the chair legs, as in *FIG. 13-1a.*

2. Place feet on the front edge of the seat. Elongate the back of your neck. Pushing with your feet, raise your buttocks slowly as high as you can pump them. Now, clasp your hands while shrugging your shoulders down onto the floor and away from your neck, making sure your elbows are in as close as possible. Make sure your cervical spine is off the floor. Keep the buttocks lifting away from the chair, as in *FIG. 13-1b.*

3. Make sure you have mastered the above before going on. With your hips still high, I want you to unlace the hands, bend at the elbows, and place your wrists onto your waist with hands cupping the buttocks. Now lower your buttocks as if to sit on your hands. You are now actually sitting on your hands with all the weight on your wrists and elbows, as in *FIG. 13-1c.*

4. When you feel balanced, rotate your hands, tipping your pelvis as you raise your left leg, as indicated in *FIG. 13-1c.*

5. Extend the chest to the chin as you raise the right leg, maintaining the slight rotation in the hip, balancing now as in *FIG. 13-1d.*

6. Inhale as you elongate the sternum, and exhale as you tighten the kneecaps and extend the heels. Breathe like this for 5 rounds, maintaining a balance with your toes just above the eyes.

7. Slowly come down as you went up, and relax.

### TIPS

1. As in FIG. 13-1b, do no push so far that it hurts the neck. It is the lift in the hips we are striving for.

2. I know this is difficult for you if you have weak wrists, but really concentrate on the inward rotation of the hips to adjust your balance.

3. When you can do this without leaning onto your neck, you are ready to do the Half Shoulder Stand from the Plough position without the chair.

### BENEFITS

Aids circulation.

Very good for varicose veins.

Helps avoid and relieve hemorrhoids.

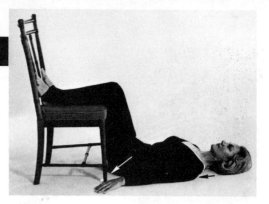

**FIG. 13-1a**

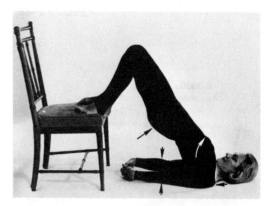

**FIG. 13-1b**

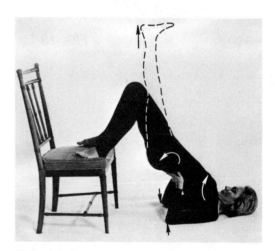

**FIG. 13-1c**

**FIG. 13-1d**

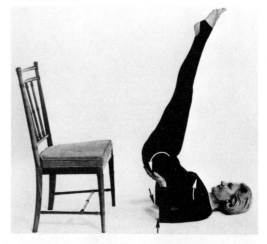

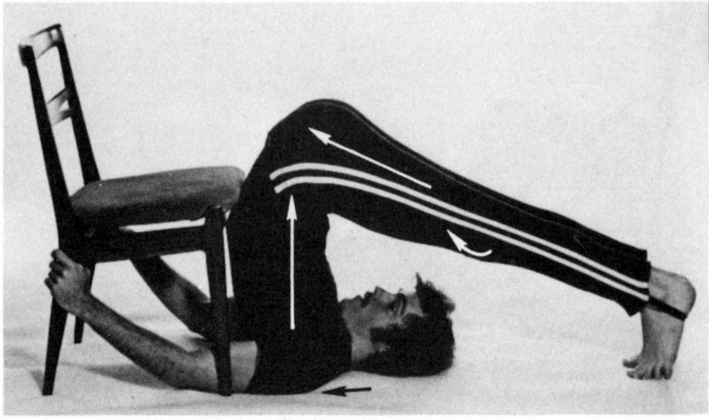

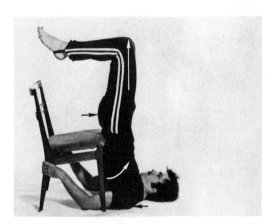

**FIG. 13-2a**

**FIG. 13-2b**

*TECHNIQUE*

1. Get into the same position as you did for the Half Shoulder Stand in *FIG. 13-1a (p. 103).*

2. Holding onto the back legs of the chair, lift yourself into the Plough position. When your toes have reached the floor, slide your arms between the chair legs. Grasp the back legs and pull the chair toward you until it touches the back of your spine, as in *FIG. 13-2a.* This will help you to sustain a Blade Squeeze.

3. Remember, we do not lean onto the neck. Straighten and elongate the spine by lifting the ischium bones toward the ceiling.

4. Holding the chair against your back, bend both knees to the forehead. Inhale while elongating, and exhale as you tighten the buttocks and raise the knees toward the ceiling, as in *FIG. 13-2b.* Take another round of breathing as you work the blades closer together recessing the spine from the floor.

5. Inhaling, keep the neck free by not bringing the chin to the chest, but extend the sternum toward the chin while lifting up. As you exhale, straighten the legs by tightening the kneecaps and elongating the heels, as in **FIG. 13-2c.**

6. When you have mastered the above and find it comfortable, you may work so your spine becomes independent of the chair.

7. While still in the **FIG. 13-2c** position, bend your elbows and work your hands to your back. Now as you continue to lift your body, work your hands into and up the back, as in **FIG. 13-2d.** With each progression of the hands into a firm supporting position as high as possible toward the shoulder blades, move the skin of the neck and shoulder area out of the way in the direction of the waist, so that the hands ultimately grip a taut back (remember how the scalp moves).

8. Inhale as you extend the sternum, exhale as you tighten the buttocks and reach the heels toward the ceiling, finding your perfect balance.

9. Slowly come out as you went into it. Take some deep breaths and relax.

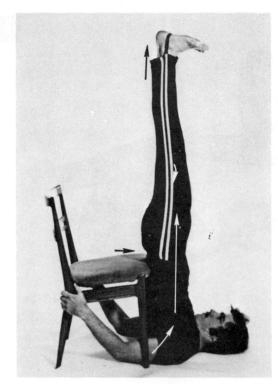

**FIG. 13-2c**

*TIPS*

**1.** It is imperative that you continually lift up for your balance, rather than let the chair push you. The main purpose of the chair is to keep your elbows in close while applying a perfect blade squeeze.

**2.** If you find the chair coming off the floor, place your hands further up the back leg of the chair to get better leverage.

*BENEFITS*

Aids asthma, bronchitis and throat ailments caused by faulty circulation.
Equalizes the thyroid and parathyroid.
Good for prolapsed organs.

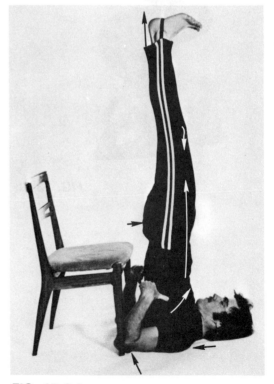

**FIG. 13-2d**

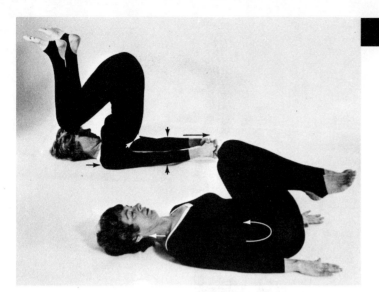

**FIG. 13-3a**

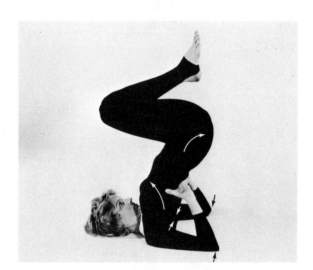

**FIG. 13-3b**

### TECHNIQUE

1. Lie flat on your back, hands at your side, with palms down, taking a few nice deep breaths.

2. Exhaling, tip your pelvis as you bend at the knees, bringing your thighs to your chest, as in **FIG. 13-3a** (right). Take 2 more breaths.

3. Press the palms onto the floor, exhaling as you push to lift the hip up, bringing knees to forehead, as in **FIG. 13-3a** (left).

4. Now, breathing normally with arms straight, *chin tucked in*, interlock your fingers. With a slight tilt from side to side, squeeze your shoulder blades together, working your elbows in as far as you can while shrugging your shoulders down toward the floor and away from the ears, as the arrow indicates in **FIG. 13-3a** (left). This will elongate the neck and lift the spine from the floor.

5. Without moving the elbows, bend the arms, placing hands onto back and close to the shoulder blades. Lift your skin as you work your hands higher up the back. Inhaling, elongate the sternum. Exhale, raising hips and thighs while concaving the back, and continue to work hands further up the back, as in **FIG. 13-3b.** Note the hand position.

6. This Step 5 is vital in order to achieve proper balance. You should have no excessive pressure on the back of the head; all the weight is supported by your arms and shoulders along with the lift you are creating with each exhalation. If any of your cervical vertebrae (neck) are pressing uncomfortably on the floor, you have not made a tight enough squeeze with your blades, nor created the proper lift while you worked your back skin up with your hands. While doing all this, you should be inhaling as you extend the sternum, and exhaling while concaving your back and reaching your ischium bones toward the ceiling. Repeat this breathing rhythm 2 times before raising knees.

7. Tighten your buttocks as you exhale, while raising your knees to the ceiling, making your thighs perpendicular to the floor. Inhaling, extend your sternum, working your hand still further onto the back as the chest touches the chin. Exhaling, tighten the buttocks as you lift high with the hips and knees, as in *FIG. 13-3c.* Do not lean *onto* your neck. Work *away*.

8. You are now ready to straighten your legs. Inhale as you elongate, extend the sternum, then tighten the buttocks and straighten the legs. Exhale, lifting tall, as you raise your kneecaps and extend, keeping your body perpendicular to the floor and your heels high, as in *FIG. 13-3d.* Stay in this position for 5 minutes with even breathing. If uncomfortable, come down into the Plough position and roll your spine down one vertebra at a time, using your hands as brakes. Bend knees to chest and lower legs.

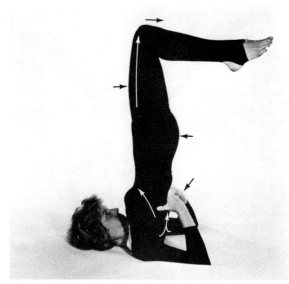

**FIG. 13-3c**

## TIPS

1. The inner effort is not visible in this posture, and it is this continual lift you experience from within your body. To understand this, have someone place a light book between your feet, and try to hold on while lifting up. The body is fully aware, and, at the same time, there is a wonderful balance.

2. I know in the beginning there is a tendency for the legs to swing out of the perpendicular position. To correct this, tighten the buttocks and rear thigh muscles while stretching up vertically.

3. Make sure you stretch your shoulders away from the neck, and bring the elbows in as close as you can within the width of your shoulders. The neck must be straight, with the chest working toward the center of the chin.

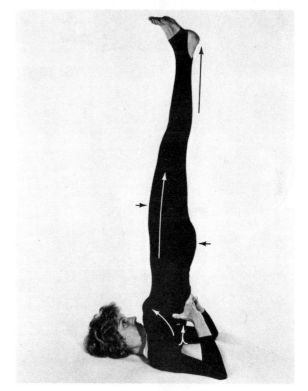

**FIG. 13-3d**

## BENEFITS

Normalizes the thyroid by stimulation

Improves circulation, benefiting brain, breathlessness, bronchitis and asthma.

Refreshes and stimulates all the internal organs and glands.

Relaxes legs and helps vein and artery conditions.

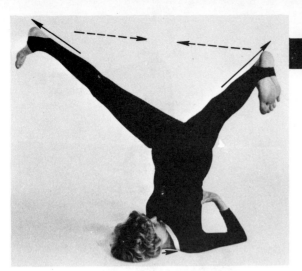

FIG. 13-4a

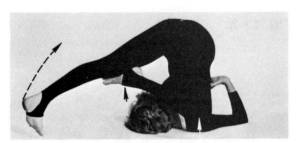

FIG. 13-4b

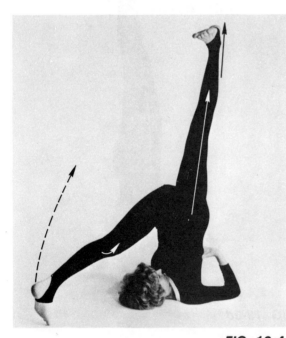

FIG. 13-4c

FIG. 13-4d

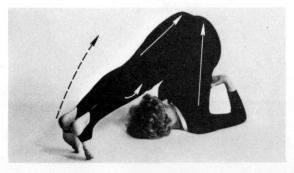

## TECHNIQUE

1. Before you begin these variations, make sure you can do the basic Shoulder Stand without any undue strain.

2. Assume the basic Shoulder Stand pose. Make sure you carry your weight on your shoulders (hence the earned name—*not* a "Neck Lean").

3. In the Shoulder Stand, maintaining a lift within the spine, exhale while splitting the legs simultaneously to the sides, extending your heels, as in **FIG. 13-4a.** Exhale as you tip your pelvis and bring legs together.

4. From the Shoulder Stand, place the top of your right foot in front of your left thigh. Exhaling, open the right knee out to the side. Tip your pelvis, and lower the left leg slowly to the floor, resisting with your right knee, as in **FIG. 13-4b.** Inhale as you lead with the right leg, raising your left leg. Exhaling, bring both legs up to meet.

5. From a perfect Shoulder Stand, maintain the proper lift throughout this pose. Ready! Inhale as you lift up with your right heel. Exhale, pulling the tummy in as you lower the left leg to the floor, as in **FIG. 13-4c.** Keep your hips centered. Lower the left leg only to the point where you can maintain the straight lift position of the right heel. In due time you will get to the floor. Inhaling, raise the left leg back up to meet the right leg. Repeat with the other leg.

6. Return to a perfect Shoulder Stand. Inhaling, lift up. Exhale as you tip your pelvis and lower both legs at the same time, as in **FIG. 13-4d.** You are bending from the hips, not leaning into the neck, as you concentrate on keeping the ischium bones high. Inhaling, keep your tummy in, and raise both legs parallel to the floor. Then exhale the remaining way up to a straight Shoulder Stand.

7. Lower yourself as in the Shoulder Stand.

## TIPS

1. I did not mention the frequency of each of these variations because you can do them separately several times or in a series.

2. Throughout these variations it is important to keep your hips centered and maintain the lift in the hips.

## BENEFITS

Strengthens the abdomen.
Develops coordination.
Helps regulate thyroid gland.

### TECHNIQUE

1. Get into the Plough position with an elongated, straight back. Clasp your hands behind you, creating a good shoulder blade squeeze with straight elbows. Inhale as you raise both legs up to a 90° angle, then exhale as you bring yourself up into a Shoulder Stand. Keep extending to get straighter, as in **FIG. 13-5a.** Restore rhythmic breathing, inhaling while elongating, and exhaling while extending heels throughout this posture.

2. After finding the proper balance, bring the hands over the head, as in **FIG. 13-5b.** Do not bend at the waist. Tighten the buttocks, and keep pumping up and lifting straighter.

3. When you have mastered the two previous Shoulder Stands without a sag in the back, you are completely balanced from within and do not need your hands. Bring them up alongside the thighs. I do not mean holding onto the thighs but just resting there. See **FIG. 13-5c.**

4. For the Pose of Tranquility, you lower the legs and place your hands where you maintain a balance, resting your leg in your hands as in **FIG. 13-5d.**

5. Exhale, and lower the legs, with control, into the Plough position and slowly roll out.

### TIPS

1. The elongated straight body is constantly leaning into the chin, but you must keep the neck relaxed. Make sure that you apply a reaching high, lifting feeling thoughout so as not to feel pressure in the head.

2. Make sure you are not feeling pressure in your cervical vertebrae. If so, shrug your shoulders further onto the floor to take the weight from the spine (hence the name "Shoulder Stand").

### BENEFITS

Excellent for tipped uterus.
Stimulates the thyroid gland.
Tones and soothes the nervous system.

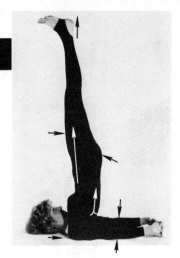

**FIG. 13-5a**

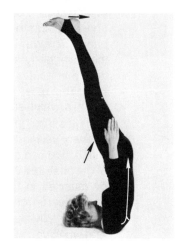

**FIG. 13-5b**

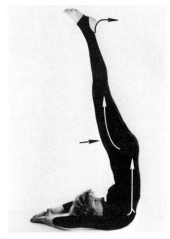

**FIG. 13-5c**
**FIG. 13-5d**

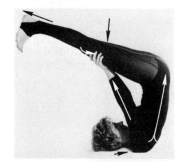

# 14 BACKWARD FLEXIBILITY OF THE SPINE

The human body stands erect because its muscles are attached to the spine and this allows man to maintain his unique posture. By acting as guy-wires, the muscles attached to the shaft of the spine pull and tug it, so that man can stand upright, bend forward or backward, sway to the sides, dance, or perform the myriad actions of a lifetime. It is very important to recognize the above concept and to tie it in to the theme of bodily interdependency which recurs on these pages. The way in which you use your upper body determines the way in which the lower body responds. Therefore, some knowledge of the spinal musculature is helpful.

The most important attached muscle is the erector spinae or sacro-spinalis, which supports the spine from the rear. It starts at the base of the spine and runs a complicated and many-branched course to the top, attached as it is to every vertebra and rib along the way. Without it, your spine would be jelly; with it, you can pull upward and backward from the floor as we will do in some of the postures that follow. From other directions, the spine is guyed up mainly by muscles in the shoulders, chest, and sides. Remember again how the body's parts function together. Whenever you exercise to strengthen back muscles, you also strengthen muscles of the front and sides (and vice versa!). And when you align your legs properly, your back goes into place. The reverse of this is true also.

Looking at this group of Postures, it might seem that they would cause or reinforce a sway back. On the contrary, they will help you to attain your natural spinal curvature, flattening the back where it formerly "swayed" and eliminating the bump of round shoulders. However, in order to reach this goal, you must pay close attention to lower-body alignment and application of the elongation and extension. This is particularly important if you have a weak-

INCORRECT

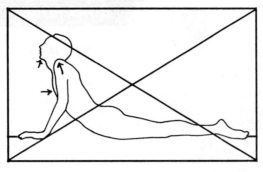

CORRECT

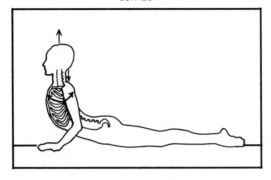

A. Deltoid
B. Trapezius
C. Latissimus Dorsi
   broadest of back muscle
D. Erector Spinae
   erector of spine
E. Gluteus Medius
   middle buttock muscle
F. Gluteus Maximus
   largest buttock muscle
G. Biceps Femoris
   tow-headed thigh

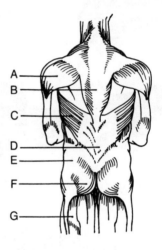

ness, for a vulnerable area is the first to tense, misalign, and become aggra-
vated. A spot that you "favor" needs gentle but persistent work.

It is difficult to describe a feeling in words, but you will find that by
extending the sternum and elongating, you will feel a lift from the lumbar
region. Your goal is to combine this with a concave backbone so that you will
experience a lift from within the entire length of the spine. Strive for this feeling
in all these postures. It will come with time and practice.

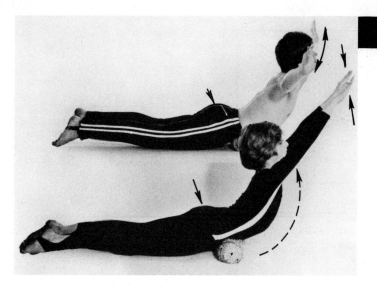

FIG. 14-1a

## TECHNIQUE

1. Roll your towel up into a firm roll or use a small hard pillow. Place it under your hips as you lie face down.

2. To raise arms, place pillow slightly above hip bone. Inhale, tighten buttocks, then exhale as you raise outstretched arms, chest and ribs from the floor, as in **FIG. 14-1a.** Take in one more breath, raising the sternum, and exhale, lifting up higher. Slowly come down, reaching outward.

3. Repeat the above procedure, but begin and end with your arms only shoulder distance apart, as in **FIG. 14-1a** (bottom). But if you find it too difficult, you may hold arms further apart, as in **FIG. 14-1a** (top). Repeat breathing pattern one more round. Then, reaching outward, slowly come down.

4. Place the pillow slightly below the hip bones so it will be easier to raise your legs. Inhale, tighten buttocks, then exhale as you raise your legs up high, together or apart, as in **FIG. 14-1b.** Your chin remains resting on your hands, and shoulders are relaxed. Take in one more breath, then exhale as you work to lift even higher. Slowly come down.

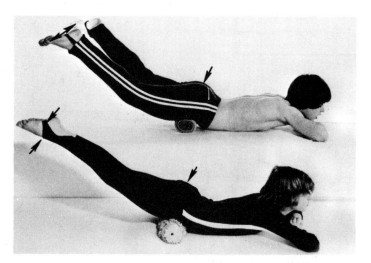

FIG. 14-1b

5. Place the towel slightly above the hip bone. Inhaling, clasp your hands behind. Exhaling, shrug shoulders back, creating a shoulder blade squeeze as you arch up, reaching with your hands toward the feet, lift the top of your head toward the ceiling. Relax the neck. Do not make this a back bend, but an elongation of the whole spinal column *(FIG. 14-1c)*.

6. Remove your pillow, so you can properly raise both your arms and legs at the same time. Take one complete deep breath before you start. Inhale; then exhale as you thrust your legs, arms and shoulders up as high as you can, as in *FIG. 14-1d*. Take one more deep breath within this position and then come down slowly.

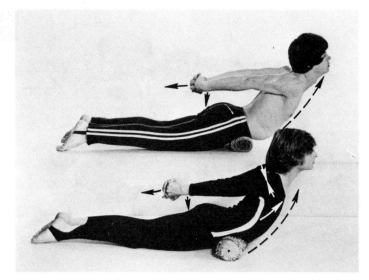

**FIG. 14-1c**

### TIPS

1. When raising arms, work so they stay in line with your ears. Do not drop your head.
2. If you can accomplish these movements with ease, you may work the arms or legs together while up in the raised position.
3. Once you have mastered the above variations, you may remove the pillow altogether and repeat the same routine. Do not be concerned if you only come up 6 inches from the floor. It is enough to get these results.

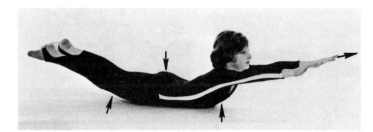

**FIG. 14-1d**

### BENEFITS

Stretches and realigns the vertebrae.

Reduces excess weight and greatly strengthens, develops, and streamlines the legs, thighs, buttocks, and shoulders.

Stimulates vital organs and glands.

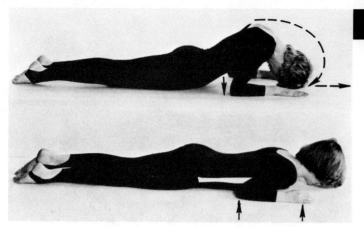

FIG. 14-2a

### TECHNIQUE

1. Lie face down. Place your arms and hands so that the elbows and palms will be flat on the floor next to the body, as in *FIG. 14-2a* (bottom).

2. Exhaling, press elbows onto the floor as you raise your chest. Tuck in your chin so as to bring your hairline on the mat, stretching the back of the neck so as to look at your navel, as in *FIG. 14-2a* (top).

3. Proceed, while inhaling and stretching forward, to drag forehead, nose, and chin forward on the mat. Pause to exhale, resting chin on the mat, as you relax the shoulders, as in *FIG. 14-2b* (bottom).

4. Inhaling, lift the head, pressing the elbows onto the floor, with eyes looking straight ahead. You pull forward with your hands as you create a creeping forward motion in your body, (like scalp motion), but do not slide, as in *FIG. 14-2b* (top).

5. Continue to inhale as you lift your ribs up, while pulling your shoulders back and away from the ears. Pull forward as you go up, tightening your buttocks.

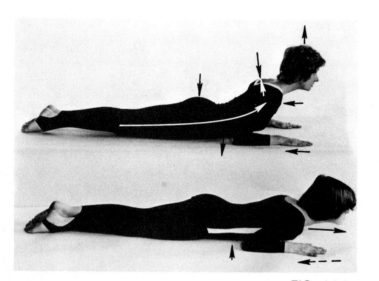

FIG. 14-2b

6. Exhale as you shrug your shoulders back, elongating the neck. Your elbows remain bent and close to your body, as in *FIG. 14-2c.*

7. Inhale again, pulling with your hands, and lift up further as if your sternum were being pulled from the top of the head.

8. On your way down, exhale as you lead with the extended sternum, maintaining a blade squeeze in back and reaching out and stretching forward on your way down, as in *FIG. 14-2d.*

9. Take 2 complete breaths before you go up 2 more times.

10. For a more advanced move, cross your legs into Lotus position. Proceed as above, and work to lower your hips to the floor.

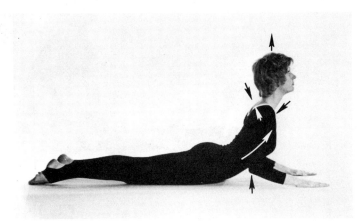

**FIG. 14-2c**

*TIPS*

1. Do not brush lightly over this creeping motion. It is very important. You are trying to crawl forward, but only moving from within your skin.

2. Make sure to keep your elbows bent and close to the body with shoulders down and back, away from the ears.

3. Keep your legs together; however, if you have trouble with your back, open legs hip-distance wide and keep the buttocks tight throughout. Hands can also be put a bit forward, in line with cheeks or higher.

4. Your hips should remain on the floor. If they will not, slide your hands out front a little.

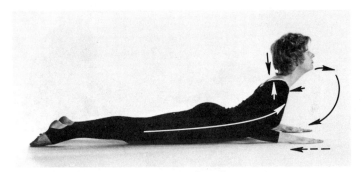

**FIG. 14-2d**

*BENEFITS*

Stimulates, massages, and relaxes all the vertebrae.
Firms bust, neck, and chin.
Firms and strengthens arms and buttocks.

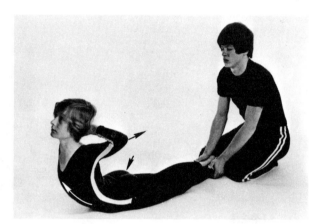

FIG. 14-3a

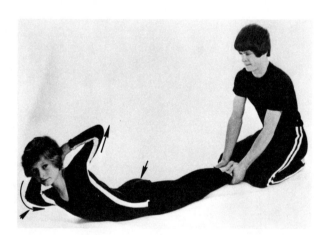

FIG. 14-3b

FIG. 14-3c

FIG. 14-3d

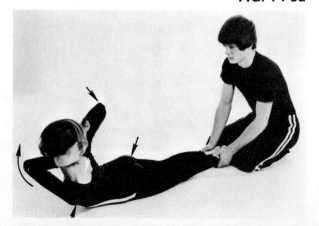

## TECHNIQUE

1. To warm up, lie face down with your feet held under something that will not lift. Chin on the floor, interlock your fingers and shrug your shoulders down away from the ears, making a tight Blade Squeeze.

2. Inhale first. Then as you exhale, tighten your buttocks, and roll up, lifting your head, chest, and ribs while working your clasped hands back toward your feet, as in **FIG. 14-3a.**

3. Still up there, inhale, extending your sternum and elongate your neck. As you exhale, work up a little higher, reaching hands further. Inhale once more and, finally, you can work your way down by exhaling, reaching forward with the ribs, sternum and chin. Relax.

4. Now you are ready for the Cobra Twist. Place your chin in on the mat and interlace your fingers, cupping the back of the head. Inhale first; then as you exhale, tighten your buttocks, and roll up, lifting first your elbow, then chin, chest and ribs. Inhale as you lift up higher, making a tighter shoulder blade squeeze. Exhale, increasing your elongation and working those elbows way back, as in **FIG. 14-3b.**

5. Inhale up once again. This time, exhale while you twist your body to the left, bringing your right elbow toward the left, and working your left elbow back and up high. Remember to keep your elongation and do not let your right elbow touch the floor, as in **FIG. 14-3c.**

6. Inhale again in up position, and bring yourself up to the center as in **FIG. 14-3b.** Do not give up! Repeat the same to the right side, as in **FIG. 14-3d.**

7. Slowly extend the chin forward as you come down. Relax when you are through. You deserve it.

## TIPS

1. It does not matter whether you use a piece of furniture or have someone hold your feet down, as long as your feet do not lift from the floor.

2. Do not be too concerned if you do not get up very high. What you are doing is important for *you*.

3. If your elbows touch the floor when you twist, practice Step 4, FIG. 14-3b until your back is stronger.

BENEFITS

Aligns the spine.
Firms buttocks and thighs.
Strengthens the shoulders.

## COBRA SALUTE

### TECHNIQUE

1. Lie face down on the mat. Place the right hand palm down, directly under the face, as in *FIG. 14-4a.* The left arm is pressed against the left ear, hand reaching out as far as it can go.
2. Inhale first. Exhale as you rise up onto the elbow, as in *FIG. 14-4b,* reaching high, keeping the left arm by the ear.
3. Continue to reach high as you raise up onto the palm of the hand, as in *FIG. 14-4c.* While still up there, inhale, elongating the spine and arm. Then exhale into a higher salute. Inhale once again, then exhale coming down slowly, extending your sternum forward and really reaching out in front with your arm, as in *FIG. 14-4d.* Then rest, as in *FIG. 14-4a.* Repeat, reversing sides.

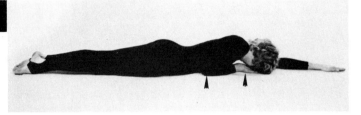

**FIG. 14-4a**

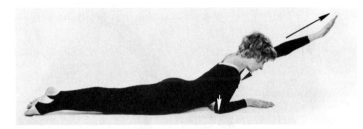

**FIG. 14-4b**

### TIPS

1. In order to get proper balance, you must have the hand directly under the face, with the nose on the knuckles. If you have weak wrists, you may place the hand further forward.
2. After you have placed your hand in the proper position, work the elbow in under the body as much as possible.
3. As you go up, concentrate on elongating your back. This will take some of the burden from the arm.

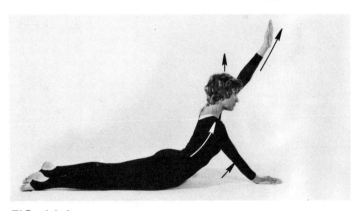

**FIG. 14-4c**

**FIG. 14-4d**

### BENEFITS

Makes the spine more supple.
Strengthens the arms.
Develops inner balance.

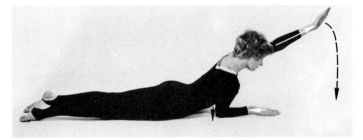

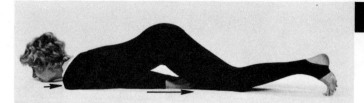

**FIG. 14-5a**

### TECHNIQUE

1. Make a fist with each hand. Place hands together, thumbs on top. Note how your hands will be as you place them under your body.

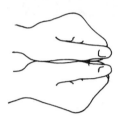

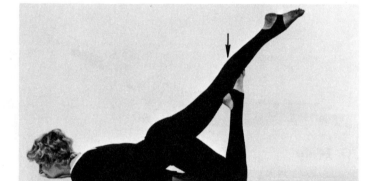

**FIG. 14-5b**

2. Lie on your stomach, applying the above hand grip with the thumbs against the floor. Tuck your arms under you and reach down as low as you can, working your forearms between your hip bones (see **FIG. 14-5a**).

3. Lower yourself on the arms. Inhale, pushing the arms and hands onto the floor. This will give you the leverage you need to raise the lower part of the body up from the floor into a nice arch.

4. To warm up, exhale as you tighten the buttocks and lift your right leg, pointing the toes. Inhale as you bend the left leg at the knee, and place the left foot over the right knee.

5. Exhale as you relax in this position, **(FIG. 14-5b).** Then come down and repeat this Locust warm-up on the other side.

6. We are now ready for the Half-Locust. Repeat Steps 1–3. Exhale as you tighten the buttocks, and raise the right leg with toes pointed (FIG. 14-5c).

7. While you are up there, inhale again and make sure you do not turn. Drop the left hip to keep the hips even. Exhale and reach outward as you slowly lower the leg. Take 2 breaths and repeat on the other side.

8. Now for the Full Locust. Repeat Steps 1–3. Exhale as you tighten the buttocks. Thrust both legs simultaneously up from the floor, with legs fully extended and touching each other at the thighs, knees and ankles (FIG. 14-5d).

9. Inhale once again, then exhale as you continue to work your arms onto the floor, while raising your thighs to come away from your hands. Slowly come down, pull the arms from under you, and relax in the Fetal position. Done properly, this is a job well done.

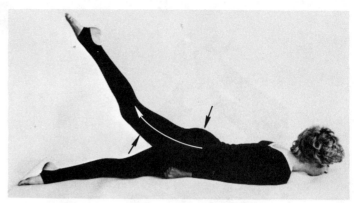

FIG. 14-5c

*TIPS*

1. The secret of this whole posture is the placement of your hands and arms between your hip bones and the pressure you apply onto the floor with your arms.

2. It is helpful to take 2 complete breaths before going into this posture. This will give you added momentum.

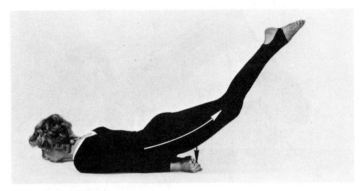

FIG. 14-5d

*BENEFITS*

Strengthens the muscles of the lower back, abdomen and thighs.
Brings a fresh supply of blood to the brain.
Firms and strengthens the arms.

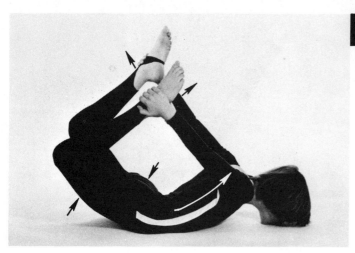

FIG. 14-6a

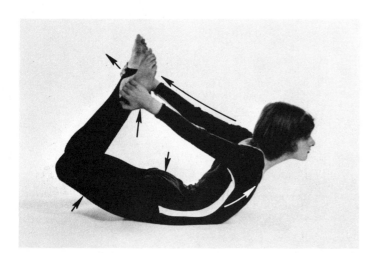

FIG.14-6b

### TECHNIQUE

1. Lie on your stomach with your chin on the mat. Grasp the arches of your feet with both hands, while knees are hip-distance apart.
2. Inhale, extending the sternum. Exhaling, shrug your shoulders back away from the ears to make a tight shoulder blade squeeze. Keep chin down. Inhale again, then exhale, tightening the buttocks as you spring your feet upward with your arms taut, creating a bow-string effect *(FIG. 14-6a)*.
3. Inhale, extending the sternum. Exhale as you raise the head, elongating the neck, lifting your chest and ribs from the floor *(FIG. 14-6b)*. Think of a "seahorse."
4. Make sure you keep your feet and knees hip-distance apart and do not drop the knees to get the head high. Keep the knees up there. Keep that lift. I do not want any "flat tire." Pressing the ankles onto the hands will help get the thighs higher.
5. Inhale once again, then exhale as you work both your head and knees high by the springing action of your shoulders, arms, hands, thighs, and ankles. They all work simultaneously. Use this breathing pattern for 2 more rounds, continuously lifting higher.

6. Once you have mastered the above, you may slowly roll on the right side, bringing your head and shoulders to the floor *(FIG. 14-6c)*. Arch on the inhalation, and roll to the side on the exhalation. To help you roll over, ease the arch slightly. When over, press knees and arches together for a stronger arch.

7. To roll back, raise left leg up high *(FIG. 14-6d)*. The rest of the body will follow. Roll up very slowly, with control.

8. Repeat to the left side for 3 more rounds. Then slowly release, and rest in the Classic Fetal Position.

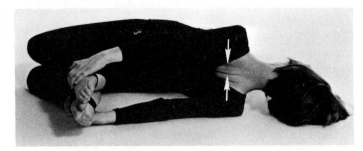

**FIG. 14-6c**

*TIPS*

1. Make sure you keep your feet and knees hip-distance apart. I know they want to open out to the side, but the stretch is not the same and is bad for your knees.

2. This should not be felt in the small of the back; if it is, you have not elongated enough.

3. For a more advanced variation, clasp your ankles and repeat from Step 1.

4. For another variation, you bring your knees and toes together and then back to hip-distance apart while in the arched bow. This gives a more advanced stretch to the thigh and further tones the buttocks.

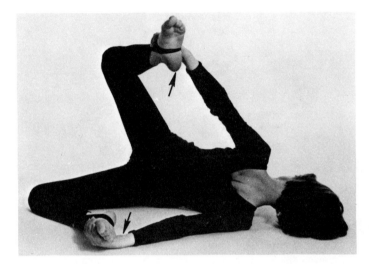

**FIG. 14-6d**

*BENEFITS*

Greatly strengthens and develops the entire spine and lumbar area.

Develops and firms muscles of the chest and bustline.

Reduces hips and buttocks.

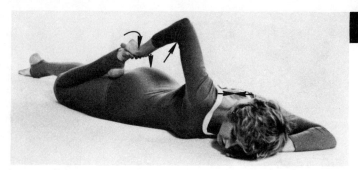

**FIG. 14-7a**

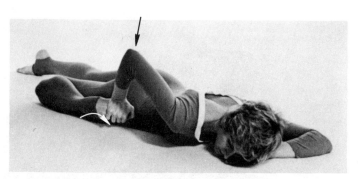

**FIG. 14-7b**

### TECHNIQUE

1. Lie down on your stomach, face turned to the left and resting on the right hand. With knees hip-distance apart, bend the left leg at the knee, keeping hip bones on the floor throughout. Take your left hand and place the toes at the wrist, grasping the instep, as in **FIG. 14-7a.** Inhale first; then exhale, as you shrug shoulders back and away from the ears. Keep the elbow high while bringing heel down to touch the buttocks, as in **FIG. 14-7a.**

2. For those of you who can reach the buttocks, continue to slide the heel down *alongside* the buttocks, toward the floor. If the heel has to leave the buttocks to go down further, you have gone too far and must backtrack to the point where the heel stays by the body. To give a little more stretch to the foot, change the hand grip, as in **FIG. 14-7b.** You inhale first, then exhale as you work the heel down. Continue this rhythm for 3 breaths. Repeat the same on the right side.

3. After you have warmed up each foot, you are going to lower both feet to the floor beside your hips, while keeping your chin on the floor, as in *FIG. 14-7c*. Take 3 breaths to work yourself into this pose; do not use force.

4. For a more advanced stretch, keep your chin on the floor and bring heels to buttocks. Keep heels on the buttocks as you inhale in shrug shoulder back position. Keep elbows up. Then exhale while you proceed to raise the knees from the floor, as in *FIG. 14-7d* (bottom). Pulling the feet toward the waist is a great help.

5. For the ultimate progression of this pose, inhale as you extend the sternum, and on the exhalation, raise the head and chest also. Now you have both the chest and knees off the floor, as in *FIG. 14-7d* (top).

6. Release your grip, come up on your knees and sit back in the Fetal Pose.

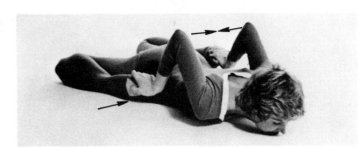

*FIG. 14-7c*

### TIPS

1. Make sure that your pelvic bones rest on the floor throughout this pose.
2. Do not let the foot spring away from the buttocks when trying to get the heel down. Keep the heel touching the body at all times, as in FIG. 14-7b.
3. Do not attempt FIG. 14-7c until you have accomplished the FIGS. 14-7a and b correctly.

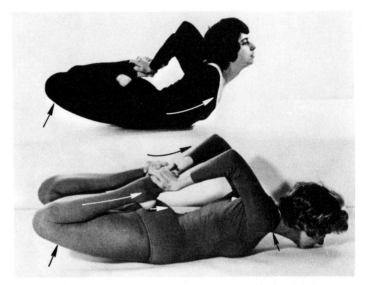

*FIG. 14-7d*

### BENEFITS

Limbers the arch and toes, helping flat feet.
Strengthens knees and stretches thighs.
Stretches shoulders and arms.

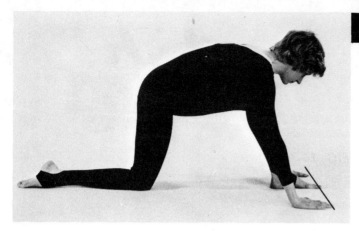

FIG. 14-8a

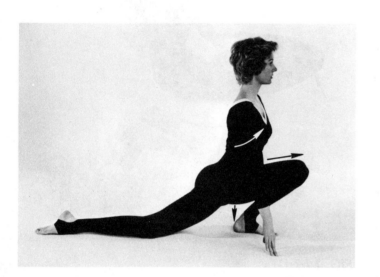

FIG. 14-8b

### TECHNIQUE

1. Kneel, extend left foot forward with the foot flat on the floor. Lower your chest onto the left thigh, placing your finger tips in line with your toes, as in *FIG. 14-8a.*

2. Inhale, then exhale, pressing the chest against the knee and pushing it forward. Drag the right leg so the left knee comes beyond the toes, but go only as far as you can while keeping the heel flat on the floor, as in *FIG. 14-8b.*

3. Keeping the knee in the extended position, place the hands on the knee and push, elongating the spine as you inhale. Extend the sternum, as in *FIG. 14-8c.*

4. Exhale as you rotate the shoulders back and down, creating a slight shoulder blade squeeze. Inhale; extend the sternum and further elongate the upper body.

5. Keeping the lift and knee forward, inhale as you raise your arms over head with palms together and thumbs crossed. Exhale as you reach higher, bringing the lift from the rib cage as in *FIG. 14-8d* (left). Keep your neck relaxed.

6. As you inhale again, it is important to maintain the upward stretch and keep the knee forward. Then as you exhale, continue the upward stretch as you arch back, looking at your fingers, as in *FIG. 14-8d* (right).

7. Keep breathing in rhythm with the motions for 3 breaths.

8. Slowly come out of the Lunge reaching upward and outward. Repeat the same with the right leg.

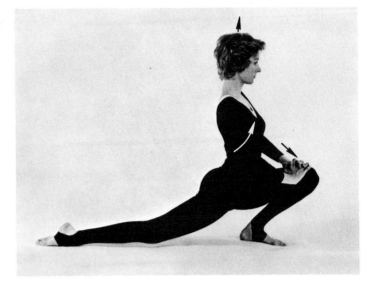

FIG. 14-8c

## TIPS

1. If you feel pressure in the lower back, you are doing this incorrectly. You are not elongating and raising the sternum enough.

2. Throughout the pose, keep the knee extended beyond the toes, with the heel flat.

3. If you would like a little more stretch in the thigh, see Step 4 and FIG. 14-8c. When you feel balanced, tighten the right knee cap and straighten the leg without lifting the hip.

4. Throughout this pose, make sure your knee remains directly over the foot.

## BENEFITS

Firms legs.
Strengthens shoulders.
Streamlines arms and upper torso.

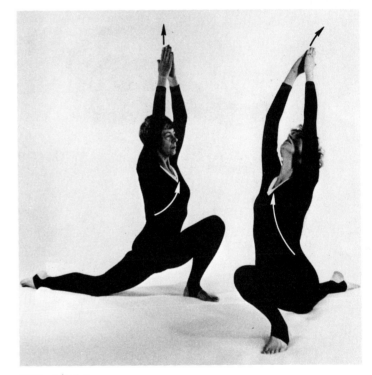

FIG. 14-8d

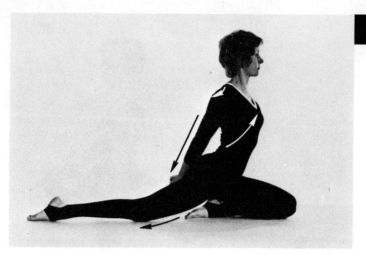

FIG. 14-9a

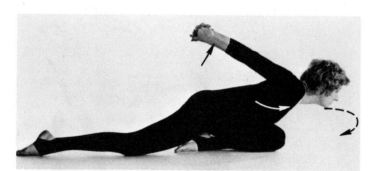

FIG. 14-9b

## TECHNIQUE

1. Kneel, slide your right leg back as you bend the left knee. Sit on your left heel. To balance, clasp your hands behind you.

2. Inhale, extending sternum as you elongate. Exhale, shrug shoulders back, creating tight shoulder blades. Squeeze with straight elbows, arms reaching downward, as in *FIG. 14-9a.*

3. Inhale, extend sternum and elongate further. Exhale slowly as you reach forward to come down, leading with the chin and sternum, as in *FIG. 14-9b.* While coming down, maintain shoulder blade squeeze and raise the arms up toward the ceiling.

Place your forehead on the floor in front of the left knee, as in *FIG. 14-9c.*

4. With forehead still on the floor, unclasp the hands; place them palms down so the elbows are in line with the shoulders and the forearms are parallel to each other.

5. Inhale; extend sternum. Exhale; raise the forehead and arms to shoulder level while creating a shoulder blade squeeze. Do not arch the neck. Keep looking at the floor, as in *FIG. 14-9d* (bottom). Take one more breath in rhythm with the motion, then come down and relax.

6. This time, keeping the arms and head down, raise your right leg from the floor, keeping it straight, as in *FIG. 14-9d* (top). Hold, then come down and relax. It is harder than it looks, is it not?

7. To come up, return your hands to the back and clasp them. Make your shoulder blade squeeze, as in *FIG. 14-9c.* Inhale, extending sternum; elongate, raising your head. Exhaling, shrug shoulders back, and to rise, lead back with your arms and shoulders. The lead in the arms will arch your back and bring you up, as in *FIG. 14-9a.*

8. Repeat on the other side, sitting on the right heel.

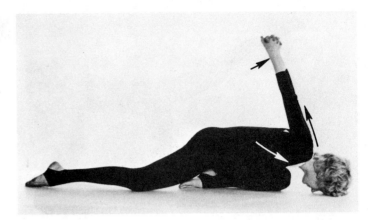

**FIG. 14-9c**

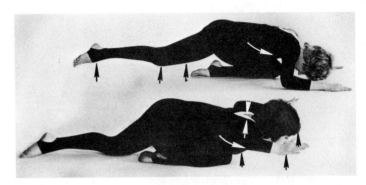

**FIG. 14-9d**

*TIPS*

1. The balance in raising and lowering the body is achieved by the elongation within the spine and the work in the arms.

2. When slowly lowering your head to the floor, do not let it fall. Keep extending the chin, then tuck the chin in, but keep the neck extension from the top of the head.

3. Throughout this posture the concentrated effort is in the shoulder blades.

*BENEFITS*

Firms thighs and buttocks.
Aids in correcting round shoulders.
Expands the chest.

127

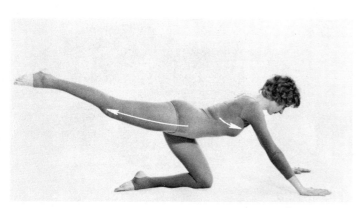

**FIG. 14-10a**

## TECHNIQUE

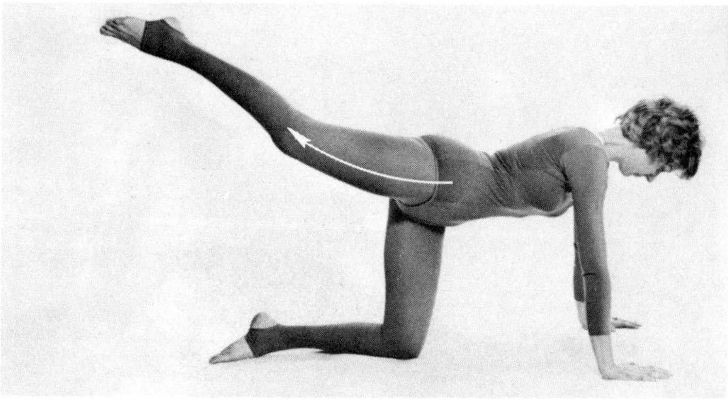

1. Place hands and knees shoulder-distance apart, so that your arms and legs are perpendicular to the floor.

2. Inhale, extend sternum. Exhale as you raise your right leg high without turning, keeping your hips level, as in *FIG. 14-10a.*

3. Inhale again. Exhale, keeping thigh high while reaching back, as in *FIG. 14-10b.* Lower your body on to the left foot, as in *FIG. 14-10c,* and relax a moment.

4. Make sure you stretch the right leg back as far as it will go.

5. Slide your body up to sit on the left heel. Place your left hand directly in front of your left knee, on the floor.

6. Inhale, extending the sternum. Exhale rotating your body until the right shoulder is in line with the right foot.

7. Inhale, lifting up, and bend your right knee, grasping the foot. Exhale, shrugging your shoulder back, elbow bent, tighten your buttocks and drop the hip, bringing your right heel to touch the buttocks, as in *FIG. 14-10d.* Turning, work the shoulders in a straight line with the knees.

8. In this position, inhale while reaching up. Exhale, working the foot closer to the buttocks. Do this for 3 rounds, and then slowly come out of it and repeat on other side.

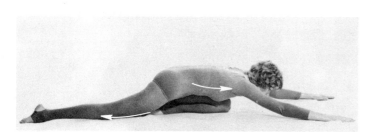

**FIG. 14-10b**

## TIPS

1. Really work to keep the thigh high while you go down, as in FIG. 14-10b. The slower you move, the better.

2. In Steps 5–7 make sure you stretch the heel back as far as it will go and also keep the hip down.

3. When you have maintained good balance, you can place your hand on the knee to get a higher lift as in FIG. 14-10d.

**FIG. 14-10c**

**FIG. 14-10d**

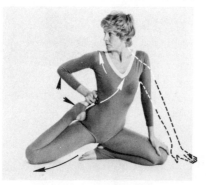

## BENEFITS

Rejuvenates the lumbar and dorsal regions of the spine.
Shoulder muscles are fully exercised.
Strengthens thighs and ankles.

### TECHNIQUE

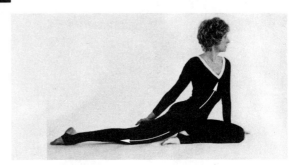

**FIG. 14-11a**

1. Kneel, slide your right leg back, placing your left foot under the right thigh, as in *FIG. 14-11a.*

2. Inhale, extending sternum, elongate the spine as you raise your right arm toward the ceiling. Exhale, shrugging your shoulder back, and at the same time, bend the right leg so the right hand will grasp the right foot.

3. Now that you have hold of your right foot, inhale, elongating the spine and extending outward with your left arm. Exhaling, bend forward at the waist and lower ribs down on your left thigh, as in *FIG. 14-11b.*

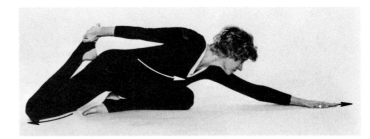

**FIG. 14-11b**

4. Inhale as you elongate the spine. Exhale as you raise your left arm, reaching outward, then raise your right knee and thigh from the floor. Again inhale, stretching tall. Exhale, springing your foot away from the body so your back will arch up, as in *FIG. 14-11c.*

5. To maintain a higher balance, inhale, once again lifting the upper body, and keep extending your hand out front. Exhale, while creating a more taut bow-string effect from shoulder to foot. Rising only as far as is possible without letting the knee touch the floor, slowly come down and repeat on the other side.

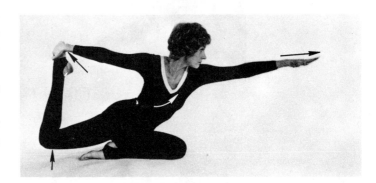

**FIG. 14-11c**

6. For this variation, just grasp the right foot with the left hand, as in *FIG. 14-11d,* and repeat Steps 1–5.

7. Reach forward with outstretched arm, to lower yourself slowly, as in *FIG. 14-11b.* Come out of this position, and repeat to the other side.

### TIPS

**FIG. 14-11d**

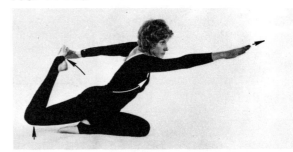

1. The right knee and thigh remain on the floor; do not sit on the foot.
2. Your balance comes from the extended lifting and pull between the outstretched arm, spine and leg.

### BENEFITS

Firms and tones the inner thigh.
Develops coordination and balance.
Stimulates circulation and increases one's vitality.

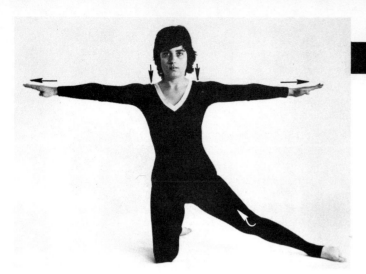

FIG. 14-12a

*TECHNIQUE*

1. Kneel on the floor with ankles together.
2. Stretch the left leg sideways out to the left and keep it in line with the right knee.
3. Turn and point the left foot, keeping the kneecap raised and in line with the foot. But keep hip facing front throughout the posture.
4. Inhale, lift your rib cage directly up as you extend the arms out sideways. Exhale as you drop the shoulders, and extend the fingers out as far as you can, as in *FIG. 14-12a.*
5. Inhale as you tighten the buttocks so that your left hip does not drop. Exhale (as you tilt your trunk) by leading with the left side of your rib cage, as in *FIG. 14-12b.* When you have gone over as far as you can, place your left hand down onto your leg.
6. Stretch up as you inhale, and raise the right arm alongside your ear. Keep extending the right arm further yet with each breath, throughout the rest of the posture.
7. Exhale as you slide the left hand down the leg as far as you can without dropping the left hip, keeping both hips facing straight forward, as in *FIG. 14-12c.* Take 3 rhythmic breaths, lifting up with each inhalation and exhalation, and extend further down the leg as in *FIG. 14-12d.*
8. To come out of this pose, inhale, reaching up tall with your right arm. Exhale and lower the arm down, and repeat the above to the right side.

*TIPS*

1. It is important to maintain a lifting up motion from the hip throughout this exercise. Do not let yourself droop or slouch.
2. Keep concentrating on maintaining both hip bones facing forward.
3. It is not how far down the leg you get that counts—it is how well aligned your body is while getting there.

*BENEFITS*

The sideways spinal movement helps stiff backs.
Pelvic region is stretched.
Keeps abdominal muscles and organs in good condition.

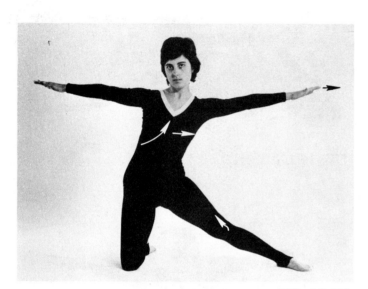

FIG. 14-12b

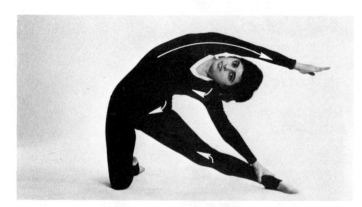

FIG. 14-12c

FIG. 14-12d

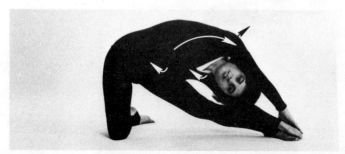

## HYDRANT POSE

### TECHNIQUE

1. Place your hands and knees in a table position. Move the right knee to the center, forming a triangle to support the body.

2. Inhale as you tuck the right knee in to touch the forehead, without foot touching the floor, as in *FIG. 14-13a.* Rotate the left hip, as this will help you lift the right hip so that you can bring your right knee out to the side and perpendicular to the hip, as in *FIG. 14-13b.*

3. Exhale, looking around the arm. Move the right knee so that it will be parallel to the floor (like a table), as in *FIG. 14-13c.* If done correctly, the foot will not be visible to you. You may take 2–3 breaths into the move to attain the correct position.

4. If you cannot do the above correctly, please do not continue, but repeat the above until your body is more flexible.

5. Inhale as you elongate your spine and lift your hip higher. Exhale as you continue to bring the right knee toward the shoulder, as in *FIG. 14-13c.* Remember not to drop the knee. Keep it level with your hip, taking 2–3 breaths to attain the position.

6. From this position, straighten out the legs, as in *FIG. 14-13d.* Extend the heel and make sure the leg is level.

7. Hold for 2 breaths and come out as you went into it. Then repeat with the left leg. When finished, rest in Fetal position.

### TIPS

1. The goal is to reach the shoulder, but only as far as you can keep the leg level.
2. Do not bend your arm or lean sideways to get that leg up.
3. The lift is from the hip and thigh.

### BENEFITS

Makes hips more flexible.
Tones the inner thigh.
Strengthens the arms.

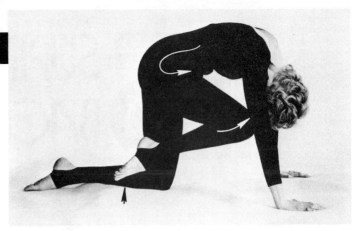

FIG. 14-13a

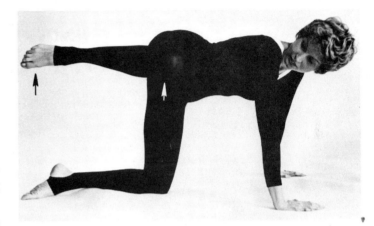

FIG. 14-13b

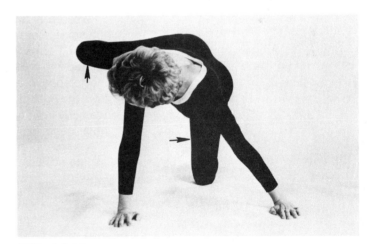

FIG. 14-13c
FIG. 14-13d

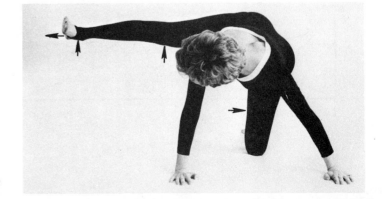

# 15 SUPINE BACKWARD FLEXIBILITY OF THE UPPER SPINE

The supine postures can be executed properly with optimum benefit by applying the "educated stretch" of the spine and torso. Very often I see students who bend only from the waistline and neck, completely disregarding the rest of the spine. Note the arched back and crunched neck in **DIAGRAM 1,** and the dangling arms, which were poorly placed because the shoulders were not rotated into a Blade. In **DIAGRAM 2,** the proper elongation and extension of the torso with accompanying concaving of the spine—wherein effort flows from the buttocks to ribs to head to buttocks with rhythmic breathing—allows the body to *lift* from within to execute a perfect Fish. There is no strain on the neck, head, or small of back. Use the "educated stretch" and proper breathing for execution of these postures so that you either start from or end with a supine position.

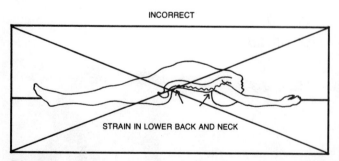

INCORRECT

STRAIN IN LOWER BACK AND NECK

**Diagram 1**

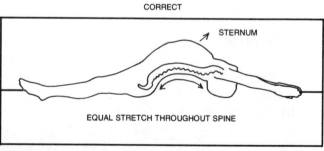

CORRECT

STERNUM

EQUAL STRETCH THROUGHOUT SPINE

**Diagram 2**

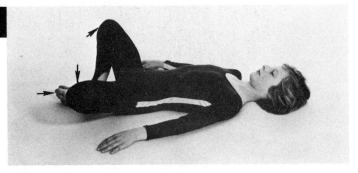

## TECHNIQUE

1. Lie on your back. Bend legs so that the heels are together and toward the crotch, with knees open and out to the side, as in *FIG. 15-1a.*

**FIG. 15-1a**

2. Place hands (palms down) under buttocks with elbows just beneath rib cage. Pressing elbows onto the floor as you inhale, lead with the sternum while arching up so the head lifts from the floor. Do not try to lift the head up. Let it hang as you slide forward. At the same time, bring shoulder blades toward the spine. Exhaling, just let your head hang down to the floor, as in *FIG. 15-1b.*

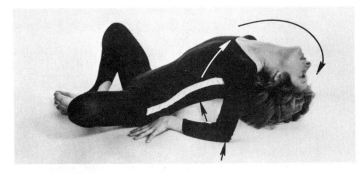

3. Inhale, raise the sternum, and elongate the neck, reaching high with the chin and leading with the chin while lifting the dorsal and lumbar regions of the spine. Do not be dependent on your elbows for that lift! Exhaling, slowly lower your head down toward the floor, as in *FIG. 15-1c.*

**FIG. 15-1b**

4. You now concentrate on taking 3 breaths. With each inhalation you lift the spine and extend the sternum, and with each exhalation you work to balance yourself at the *top* of your head.

5. When you find that comfortable balance spot on your head and are not dependent on your elbows for your lift, you can continue.

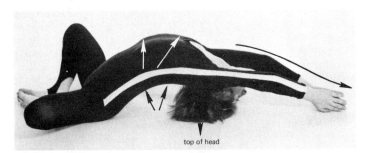

6. Without using your elbows, bring hands to the inner thighs, working your knees closer to the floor, as in *FIG. 15-1d.* Inhale to extend the spine and exhale as you press down on the thighs.

**FIG. 15-1c**

**FIG. 15-1d**

7. To come out, press your elbows onto the floor and lift, leading with the chin up high, as you elongate the neck. Raise the head, tuck the chin in as you tip your pelvis, round your shoulders, and slowly roll spine on the floor.

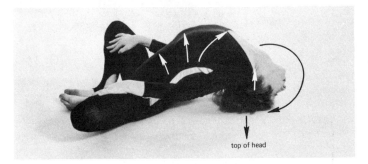

## TIPS

1. Make sure you gain your lift from arching and reaching your whole spine up, not by rolling onto the neck.

2. I cannot say enough on the importance of the lift of the sternum—from within the whole spine.

3. If you feel sick in this pose, it could be that your neck is out of alignment or there is too much pressure in the cervical area. Work to raise the chest more and concentrate on elongating the neck, only lower, as in FIG. 15-1b.

## BENEFITS

Relieves tension in neck and upper back.
Develops chest and bust line.
Alleviates asthma and respiratory complaints.

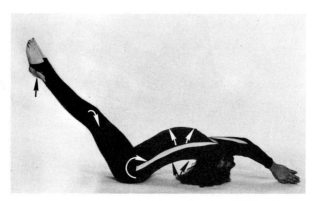

FIG. 15-2a

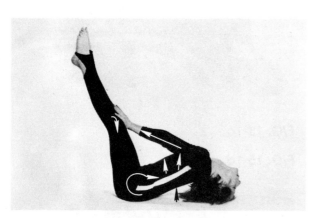

FIG. 15-2b

FIG. 15-2c

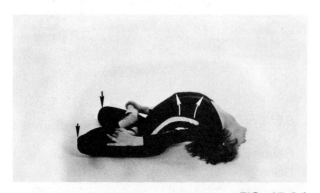

FIG. 15-2d

## TECHNIQUE

1. Before you try this Fish Pose, make sure you have accomplished the Frog Pose without pressure in the neck.
2. Lie down with legs out in front, hands under the buttocks, with elbows just beneath the rib cage.
3. Inhaling, lift your sternum, arch your spine, squeezing your shoulder blades together as you lift head from the floor. Do not tense the neck, elongate it. Exhale, reaching high with the chin; lower the top of your head to the floor. If you need more details, see the Frog Pose.
4. When you have the proper balance on the head—not the neck—and also the buttocks, you may proceed by inhaling while raising hands up, and exhaling while you lower the hands over head, as in **FIG. 15-2a.**
5. Take 3 good breaths in this pose. While inhaling you are continually maintaining the lift in the spine. When exhaling, you stretch your hands out further.
6. To raise your arm and leg, inhale first. Exhaling, tip your pelvis, raise legs up toward the ceiling, as in **FIG. 15-2b.** Inhale again as you enforce the lift.
7. Now, raise your arms up, placing hands on legs, as in **FIG. 15-2c.** Both arms and legs should be kept straight, do not bend at the knees or elbows. Hold this pose for 2 breaths; keep working on that lift. Then exhale as you slowly lower legs and arms to the floor.
8. For the Lotus Pose, cross your legs in a Lotus position and lie down. Inhale as you lift up on your head; then exhale as you work your knees to the floor, holding onto your toes, taking 3 breaths, as in **FIG. 15-2d.**
9. To come out, review Step 7 as in the Frog Pose.

## TIPS

1. It is advisable to do only one of these variations at a time, but to hold the pose for the recommended period.
2. Make sure you concentrate on keeping that lift and do not sag one iota.
3. In the Fish Pose, the trachea is expanded, so breathe deeply to ventilate fully the upper lobes of the lungs.

## BENEFITS

Keeps spine and neck supple.
Alleviates asthma.
Aids respiratory complaints.

## TECHNIQUE

1. Kneel with knees and feet hip-distance apart. Place your hands at your hips and tighten your buttocks, as in *FIG. 15-3a.* Inhale, stretching upward as you lead forward from the hips. Exhale as you shrug your shoulders back, lowering your hands to the heels (one at a time or both together) if you can. If this is too easy, clasp the ankles.

2. Inhaling, tighten the buttocks; lift up from the hips, not the shoulders. Exhale, leading further forward but only to the point where your thighs are perpendicular to the floor, as in *FIG. 15-3b.* Repeat Step 2 two more times. Slowly come up.

3. This time place your hands on the front of the thighs, tuck in chin, tip your pelvis and tighten your buttocks, as in *FIG. 15-3c.*

4. Inhale, extend your sternum; lift (from the hips and ribs) straight up, and shrug shoulders forward. Exhale as you maintain the position, and lean back as far as you can without sagging, as in *FIG. 15-3d.*

5. To come up, lead with the navel to keep the back straight. Do not arch. Repeat Step 4 two more times.

6. Relax in the Fetal Pose.

## TIPS

**1.** If you feel pressure in your lower back, you are not stretching upward enough.

**2.** As in Step 4, make sure your shoulders are shrugged forward and away from your ears. Do not hunch.

**3.** As in Step 5, make sure you do not sag on your way up. Keep a straight body.

## BENEFITS

An excellent stretch for the back and thighs.
Strengthens the neck.
Makes feet more flexible.

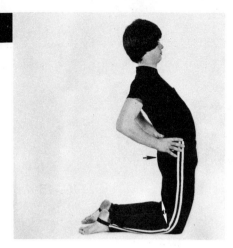

**FIG. 15-3a**

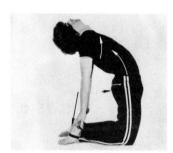

**FIG. 15-3b**

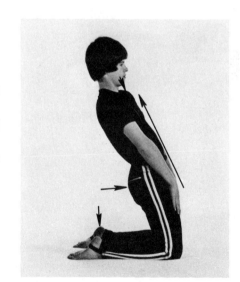

**FIG. 15-3c**

**FIG. 15-3d**

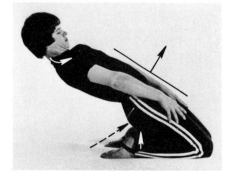

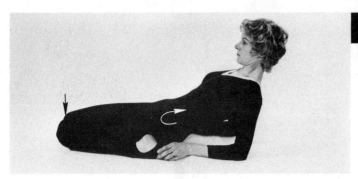

FIG. 15-4a

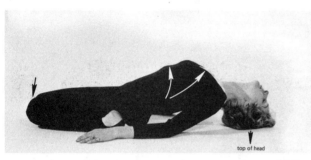

FIG. 15-4b

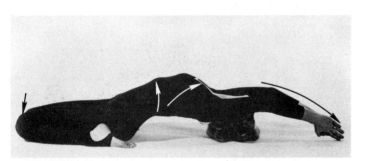

FIG. 15-4c

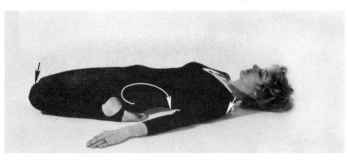

FIG. 15-4d

## TECHNIQUE

1. Sit on the floor, with legs out in front. Bend each leg to bring feet against the buttocks. Knees remain together.

2. Lean back carefully on your elbows, as in **FIG. 15-4a.** Inhale, extending the sternum, thereby creating an arch. Exhale and elongate the neck, lowering the top of the head to the floor, as in **FIG. 15-4b.**

3. Inhale, maintaining your arch. Exhale as you bring both arms overhead with palms together, as in **FIG. 15-4c.** Take 3 extending breaths while in this pose.

4. Return arms beside body, pressing the elbows onto the floor. Raise the head by leading with the chin to the chest bone. Tip your pelvis, and slowly lower the small of the back, rib cage, shoulder blade, and, finally, the head to the floor.

5. To remove the slight arch that you have, slide your hands down the buttocks toward the thigh while further tipping your pelvis. Relax in this position for a few moments. To come out, come back up on your elbows; then lift yourself up as you went into the posture.

## TIPS

1. Keep your knees on the floor at all times.
2. If this causes discomfort in your knees, place a thin cloth behind the knee before bending it.
3. Keep the arch in the spine, in order not to strain your neck.

## BENEFITS

Stimulates abdominal organs and pelvic region.
Expands the chest.
Tones legs.

### TECHNIQUE

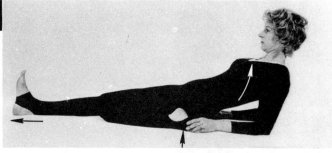

**FIG. 15-5a**

1. Sit up and bend the left leg at the knee as you bring the foot against the buttocks. Place foot beside, not under, the buttocks, as in *FIG. 15-5a.*

2. Lower the body down and rest on the elbows. Make sure you can keep the left knee down on the floor. If so, you may continue to lower the body to the floor. To reduce the arch in the back, slide the hands down under the buttocks and away while tipping, as in *FIG. 15-5b.* Make sure that you knee is still down on the floor.

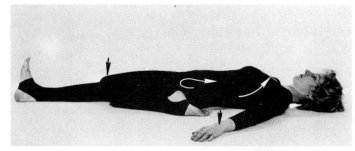

**FIG. 15-5b**

3. I want you to continue only when you can correctly accomplish the *FIGS. 15-5a* and *b.* While in this next position, attempt to tip your pelvis. Bend the right leg at the knee and interlace your fingers around the knee. Inhaling, elongate extended sternum. Exhale, pressing the left knee onto floor. Inhale again, shrugging shoulders, and exhale as you bring the right knee toward the chest, as in *FIG. 15-5c.* Take 3 breaths to ease the knee closer.

4. Come out of this position the way you went into it, and repeat, using the other side.

5. Sit up and place both feet along the thighs and slowly roll back to the floor, tipping your pelvis. Relax in this position (as in *FIG. 15-5d*) for a few moments to try to lessen the arch in your back by sliding the buttocks down and tipping your pelvis.

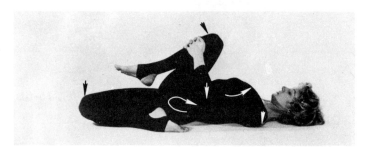

**FIG. 15-5c**

### TIPS

1. If you have difficulty bringing your foot beside the buttocks, as in FIG. 15-5a, and it is uncomfortable in the arch of your foot, do not continue with this posture, but go back and work on the Closed Bow.

2. For the majority, there will be a slight arch in your back in this posture, but try to lessen it by sliding your buttocks down and away while tipping your pelvis.

3. Throughout this whole exercise, the left knee should remain on the floor. If it comes up, you have gone too far and must work to get it down by exhaling and tipping.

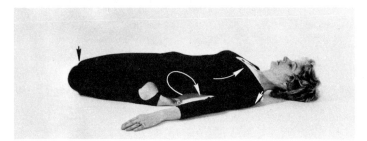

**FIG. 15-5d**

### BENEFITS

Stretches the thighs.
Makes the feet more flexible.
Makes hips more flexible.

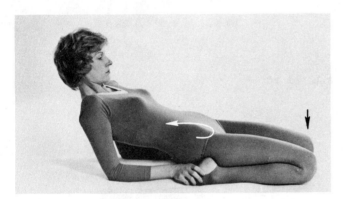

FIG. 15-6a

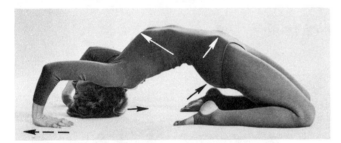

FIG. 15-6b

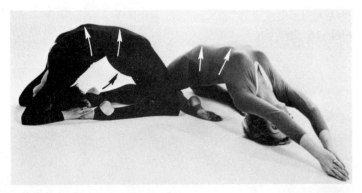

FIG. 15-6c

FIG. 15-6d

## TECHNIQUE

1. Kneel down with legs hip-distance apart and heels just under the thighs. Make sure your heels turn outward so the foot curves a little, as in *FIG. 15-6a.*

2. Lower body down on your elbows, as in *FIG. 15-6b.*

3. Lower head to the floor and place hands under shoulders, as in *FIG. 15-6c.*

4. Inhale, pressing hands onto the floor. Exhale, stretch the arms, and raise the whole body from the knees by stretching the thighs. Tighten the buttocks, stretch the entire spine, and bend the elbows as you lower top of head to the floor. Inhale once again, elongating the spine and lifting slightly. Exhale, lowering the head in closer to the feet. Place palms together over the head, as in *FIG. 15-6d* (right). No weight is on the hands. The pose is accomplished by lifting hips and thighs. Repeat the breathing rhythm for 2 more rounds as you work into a higher arch.

5. To come out of this posture, place the hands back under the shoulders, as in *FIG. 15-6c.* Lift head up, leading with the chin, and tuck the chin in toward the chest *(FIG. 15-6b).* Then tip your pelvis, lowering your ribs, shoulders, and head on the floor, turning the body to one side to move the legs out from under you.

6. More advanced students can begin the Kneeling Bridge Pose with their feet and knees together or apart, and continue with the above procedures. This posture requires a stretch within the entire spine and this is attained by stretching the neck backward, resting the top of the head on the soles of the feet, and lifting the pelvis and further stretching the thighs, as in *FIG. 15-6d* (left). To come out of this pose, see Step 5.

## TIPS

1. If your knees spring up while attempting this pose, refer to the Vise Press.

2. Be careful not to turn the head under so that the neck is bent back too far.

3. Tightening the buttocks as you lift the pelvic region will enable you to get a higher lift.

## BENEFITS

Tones up the entire spinal region.
Aids circulation and provides excellent massage for the heart.
Firms thighs and buttocks.

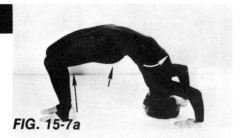

### TECHNIQUE

1. Lie down; bend your knees. Grab your ankles and bring them close to the buttocks. Place hands (palms down) under shoulders.

2. Inhale, extending sternum, and tighten buttocks. Lifting high with hip and spine as you exhale, push with your palms, coming to rest on the top of your head while arching the body, as in **FIG. 15-7a.**

3. Before going up further, check these things: 1) feet must be parallel and flat on the floor, with legs hip-distance apart, and knees directly above feet; 2) heels of your hands must be pressed onto the floor; 3) fingers must be pointing toward the feet; and 4) do not let the knees lunge beyond the toes. When all points are checked, continue.

4. Inhaling, extend sternum, and tighten buttocks. Lead with the sternum as you exhale, and push with your hands, straightening your arms while raising your head from the floor, as in **FIG. 15-7b** (left). Keep the neck relaxed.

5. At this point, adjust your balance if necessary by walking feet in closer, in order to keep your sternum in line with your hips, as in **FIG. 15-7b** (right).

6. When you have maintained balance, inhale, placing your right hand in the center. Exhale, raising your right foot to the center. Exhale; raise the left leg, as in **FIG. 15-7c.** Slowly lower it and repeat to the right side.

7. If you are still up and game, inhale, placing your right hand in the center. Exhale, raising your left hand and placing it as in **FIG. 15-7d.** Slowly lower it and repeat with the right arm.

8. To come down, it is important to move the chest toward the hands and not merely fold the leg. Tuck the chin in and carefully lower yourself to the floor.

9. Remain in this position for 3 deep Rib Cage Breaths, and relax. You have earned it.

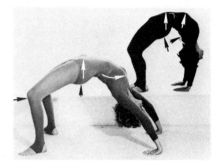

**FIG. 15-7b**

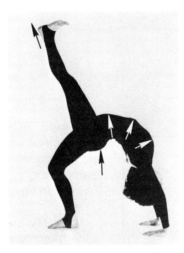

**FIG. 15-7c**

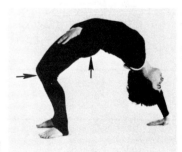

**FIG. 15-7d**

### TIPS

1. Throughout the Wheel stretch the arms from the shoulders to keep the arms straight. Also, keep your neck relaxed. Do not hunch your shoulders up by your ears; work them away.

2. You should not feel pressure in the lumbar region. If you do, you are not leading enough with the sternum.

3. The tendency is to spread the knees too far apart. If this is so, work your knees in a little towards each other, bringing them directly above the feet.

4. If you find this Pose too difficult, practice the Kneeling Bridge Pose; you can experience the lift in the body that has to be maintained so that you do not bear all the weight on your wrists.

### BENEFITS

Strengthens arms and legs.
Makes the spine flexible.
Tones abdomen and thighs.

# 16 SPINAL TWISTS

INCORRECT

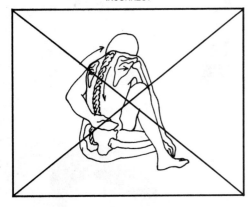

CORRECT

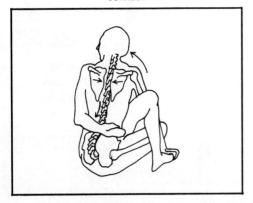

The Spinal Twist Pose requires a maximum torsion of the vertebral column (rotating one vertebra over the other throughout its length). The Twist Poses are not recommended for students with bad backs until they have correctly learned how to elongate their spines and are free from constrictions. The Twists can be applied to strengthen and align the spine once these problems have been corrected.

Rotation of the vertebral column brings energetic massage on the sensory, motor and visceral nervous roots thus revitalizing all three of those systems. In the forced twisting movements of the lumbar region, the muscles are especially stimulated, with the result that their stretching and contracting isometrically heightens distribution of blood.

As the benefits work upward, the contracted liver and spleen are toned, and cease to be sluggish.

Sprains in the shoulder, calcium deposits, or displacements of the shoulder joints are relieved and the shoulder movements become freer.

Finally, the muscles of the neck gain strength.

It is very important that you begin the Twist with the right thigh pressing against the abdomen. This will increase peristaltic action in the intestines and diminish constipation. To follow the proper peristaltic movement, the right side of the abdominal region is compressed first. Apart from the large intestine, the liver and the right kidney are stimulated during the first half of the exercise, and the spleen, pancreas, and left kidney during the second half.

Concentrate on relaxing the muscle structure in the spinal column and follow mentally the progression of the twist as it moves from the sacrum to the skull.

### TECHNIQUE

1. Kneel with right thigh, hip and shoulder against the wall; sit down. Place your feet as far away as they will go from the wall but close to the body, as in **FIG. 16-1a.**

2. Place your hands, palms to the wall, with elbows shoulder-high, as in **FIG. 16-1b.**

3. Inhale; extend sternum, lifting from the hip. Exhaling, twist to the right, as in **FIG. 16-1c.** The chin and sternum must turn together. Keep the neck relaxed, since the twist is felt in the shoulder. You are pushing with the right hand, causing the right shoulder blade to squeeze toward the center and bringing your left breast closer to the wall. Do not lose the lift on your left side; that is very important. Keep fingers still in line.

4. Inhale, extending sternum as you lift to elongate. Exhale as you twist even further, bringing your left breast to the wall. Take several deep breaths in rhythm with the twist; bring both sides of your chest even with the wall and your shoulders even and level facing the wall, as in **FIG. 16-1d.**

5. Slowly come out of Twist. Repeat Steps 1–4 with left side against the wall.

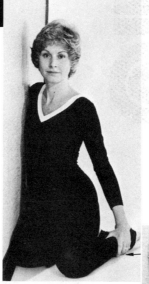

FIG. 16-1a

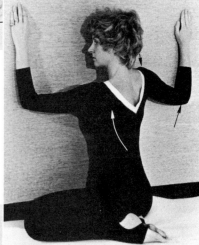

FIG. 16-1b

### TIPS

1. Make sure you lift to elongate on each inhalation and twist further on each exhalation.
2. Do not lean toward right but keep the spine straight.
3. Keep the neck relaxed.
4. The Twist originates in the lower spine and works up into the shoulder blades, not into the neck.

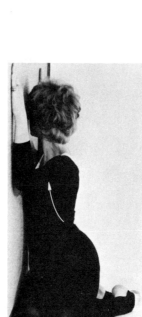

FIG. 16-1c

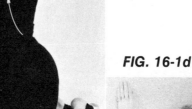

FIG. 16-1d

### BENEFITS

Excellent for round shoulders.
Slims arms, midriff, waist and hips.
Helps spine become more flexible.

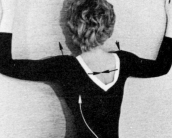

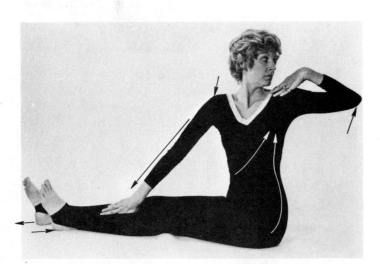

**FIG. 16-2a**

**FIG. 16-2b**

### Propped Warm-Up

*TECHNIQUE*

1. Sit tall on your ischium bones, with legs stretched out in front.
2. Place your right hand between the legs with the right palm against the right knee. Lower the hand down the leg as you twist.
3. Place your left hand directly in back of you with your wrist up against your buttocks, as in *FIG. 16-2a.*
4. Using your hand and arm for support, inhale, extending sternum as you lift up, and elongate, concaving the spine.
5. Still reaching up, exhale as you twist to the left. Starting from the hips, which will shorten the left leg, continue twisting up the rib cage, chest, and shoulders. You are creating a left-sided shoulder blade squeeze.
6. Keep your shoulders down away from your ears. Your neck is relaxed as you slowly turn it to the left.
7. Take several deep breaths in rhythm, inhaling as you lift and exhaling as you twist. Work to the point where your shoulders are parallel with the legs.
8. Slowly come out of this and repeat on the opposite side.

### Winged Warm-Up

*TECHNIQUE*

1. Repeat Steps 1–5. Once you have aligned your twist properly so that your shoulder and legs are parallel, lift the left hand and place it on your left shoulder. The upper arm and elbow must be parallel with the floor, as in *FIG. 16-2b.*
2. Repeat Steps 6–7 as you twist, keeping that elbow up.

### TECHNIQUE

1. Sit tall on your ischium bone with legs stretched out in front.
2. Bend your left knee and place the sole and heel flat on the floor, with the left ankle as close and as high up the right thigh as possible.
3. Bend your right arm, placing your right hand onto the right shoulder.
4. Inhale, as you straighten the spine. Exhale as you lead forward with your right elbow on the outside of the bent left knee. Shoulder and knee are challenging each other, as in **FIG. 16-2c.**
5. Inhale, elongating. Exhale as you remove the right hand from the shoulder, reversing the bend in the elbows. Ease the leg enough so you can bring your right hand under the leg and around at the waist. Clasp your left hand to the right, as in **FIG. 16-2d.**
6. Inhaling, extend sternum; elongate and straighten the spine. Keeping the lift, exhale as you twist the body further to the left. You are creating a left-sided shoulder blade squeeze. Your neck is relaxed as you look over the left shoulder.
7. Take several deep breaths in rhythm, inhaling to lift up, and exhaling as you twist further. Slowly come out of this position; repeat with the right knee bent up, twisting to the right.

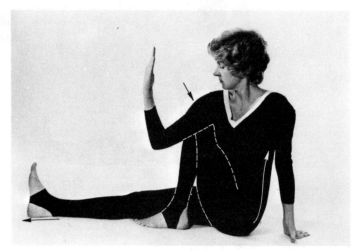

**FIG. 16-2c**

### TIPS

1. In the Warm-Ups, it is important to keep a stiff straight arm pushing against the leg for leverage.
2. As you twist the hips in the Warm-Ups, help your legs to be uneven.
3. In the One-Legged Twist, keep extending the heel, elongating the straight leg.
4. Your buttocks remain on the floor at all times.

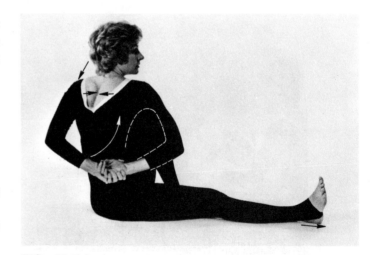

**FIG. 16-2d**

### BENEFITS

Slims the waist and midriff.
Arms and hands are strengthened.
Chest is expanded.

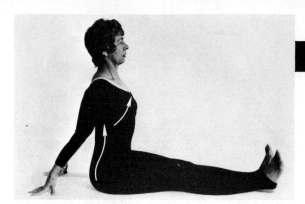

FIG. 16-3a

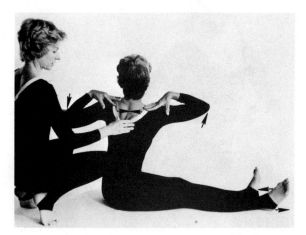

FIG. 16-3b

### TECHNIQUE

1. Sit tall with legs together. Place your hands in back of you to aid in lifting the upper body, and rotate your hips forward so you are straight up on your ischium bone (seat bone), as in **FIG. 16-3a.**

2. Inhaling, extend sternum, lifting up. Exhale as you create a shoulder blade squeeze; concave the lower back.

3. Now that your back is in the correct position, place your hands on your shoulders with upper arms parallel with the floor, as in **FIG. 16-3b.**

4. Inhale, extend sternum, lift up and keep elbows high. Exhaling, twist to the left; pull back the left elbow, hip and leg. This makes the left leg shorter than the right, as in **FIG. 16-3c** (right). Imagine my knee in your back, and press against it to straighten the spine.

5. Inhaling, extend sternum. Exhaling, squeeze out all the air and further twist to the left, creating a stronger shoulder blade squeeze. Keep the elbows high. Repeat Step 5 for 1 more breathing cycle, as in **FIG. 16-3d.**

6. Inhale, lifting tall, and return to the center. Repeat to the right side.

7. End with a forward bend on an exhalation, leading with your elbows and sternum as you reach forward with elbows. Lower your ribs onto the thighs, with elbows ending down beside the legs as you relax.

### TIPS

1. Maintain a lift from the hips, straight up within the entire upper body, twisting as one unit. *Watch* that you do not lean back. Sit tall on those ischium bones.
2. Throughout, your chin stays in line with the sternum.
3. Do not sag the lower back. Keep it concaved and maintain a lift from the hips.
4. Keep shoulders down away from
5. You know you are correct if you sense a feeling of lightness within the body.

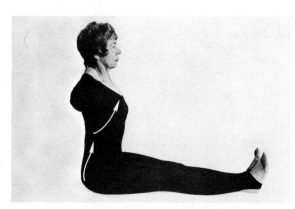

FIG. 16-3c

FIG. 16-3d

### BENEFITS

Creates good posture.
Tones the arms, midriff, waist, and hips.
Aids circulation and releases tension.

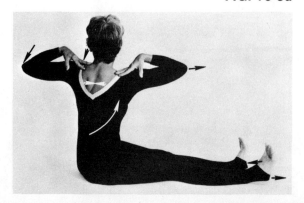

### Classic Twist

*TECHNIQUE*

1. Sit straight with legs out in front of you. Bend the left leg, and bring the left foot under the right buttock. Press the left knee to the floor.

2. Inhale as you bend the right knee, and exhale as you place the right foot to the outside of the left knee, as in *FIG. 16-4a.*

3. Inhale, elongating as you raise your left hand, and reach high toward the ceiling, stretching the whole left side of the torso. Keeping the stretch in the body, place your left hand on your left shoulder and reach out in front with the elbow, as in *FIG. 16-4b.* The shoulder is pressed against the outside of the right knee. This will bring your right knee behind the left shoulder as high as you can get it. Exhale and grasp the right instep with your left hand, as in *FIG. 16-4c.*

4. Inhale, elongating as you raise the right hand up, reaching to the ceiling to stretch the whole torso. Turn to the right, and look over your right shoulder as you shrug your shoulders back. Exhaling, lower the arm. Bend it at the elbow so that you can touch the inner thigh of the right leg with your fingertips, as in *FIG. 16-4d* (left).

5. Inhale, extending your sternum to elongate the spine. Exhale, maintaining the lift as you twist further into the position. Take several breaths in rhythm with this twist motion. Come out of this position, then either repeat to the other side or continue on.

### Knotted Twist

*TECHNIQUE*

1. For more leverage, remove the left hand from the right foot, and bring it under the right leg to grasp the right hand at the waist, as in *FIG. 16-4d* (right).

2. Repeat breathing pattern, as in Step 5.

*TIPS*

1. In FIG. 16-4b it is most important that you work the knee up in back of the shoulder as far as possible. This will enable you to get the proper grip on the foot.

2. If you are having trouble touching the inner thigh with the fingertips, check to see that you have turned properly, shoulders shrugged back, and are looking

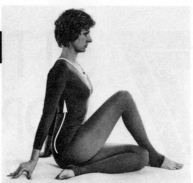

FIG. 16-4a

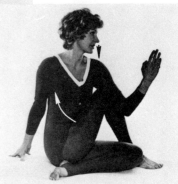

FIG. 16-4b

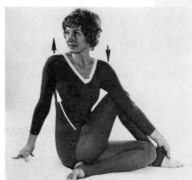

FIG. 16-4c

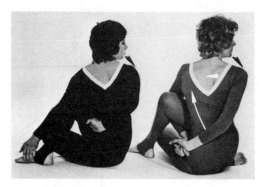

FIG. 16-4d

as far back to the opposite corner as you can. Believe it or not, you can make it!

*BENEFITS*

Massages internal organs.
Realigns vetebrae and relieves tension.
Gives a lateral pull to the pelvic region.

# 17 SITTING FORWARD BENDS

Does **DIAGRAM 1** look familiar to you? If this is the way you attempt a Sitting Forward Bend, you are putting an extreme strain on your lower spine, and more so if you forced yourself into position by bouncing or pulling yourself down. The rounded, hunched back in **DIAGRAM 1** indicates that the entire spine has been rendered very vulnerable because of its being forcibly pulled outward from its natural "concaved" position; the spine appears as a strained, bony protrusion. At the same time, imagine the oxygen-starved lungs in the sunken rib-cage, not to mention the congested abdominal organs.

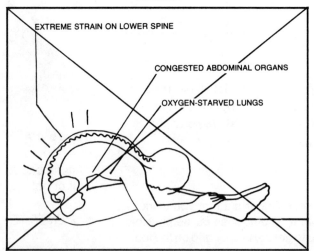

INCORRECT

EXTREME STRAIN ON LOWER SPINE

CONGESTED ABDOMINAL ORGANS

OXYGEN-STARVED LUNGS

*Diagram 1*

In executing these postures, try to imagine that you are helping your spine to attain its natural position by having your energy and effort going in several directions simultaneously. To go forward properly, as in **DIAGRAM 2,**

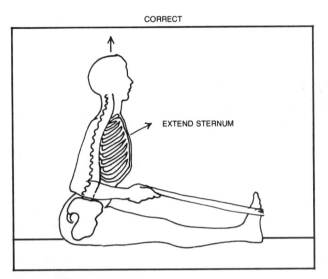

CORRECT

EXTEND STERNUM

**Diagram 2**

you first plant the ischium bones firmly beneath you, "aiming" them onto the floor. Direct your energy both down the legs to the elongated heel and back toward the rooted ischium bones. Simultaneously direct your energy upward from the ischium bones to the top of the head, then from head to floor beneath those bones, elongating the body, and extend the sternum and concave the spine so that you are well-based (the legs) and in the optimum position (elongated and concaved) before starting forward. You will find that by applying the principles of elongation and concaving upward, you will be able to utilize this natural placement of the spine to move forward and down. Use a "two steps down, one step up" rhythm—almost as if you were moving by a ratchet—as you breathe downward. The rhythm for all the following postures is: Tummy-In, inhale, elongate; then exhale and concave, moving toward the ultimate position. Go back half the distance of the move but do not lose the "ideal" back. Tummy-In, inhale, elongate, and exhale as you concave. Continue in this manner, taking as many breaths as necessary until you reach the farthest point at which you can still maintain the elongated and concaved back. Then *stop!* Relax within the posture for a few moments before taking one final breath and elongating. Exhale further into the move and surprise yourself (you went further than you thought you could).

I call this application of the elongated-extended-concaved spine an "educated stretch," and want you to use it as you pursue your goal of attaining these postures. Remember: in any of these postures, breathe in rhythm and *go only as far as you can* without losing the "educated stretch." The day will come when your persistence will pay off and you will achieve the satisfaction of completing the posture while maintaining a perfectly positioned spine and torso.

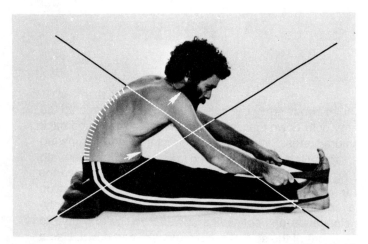

FIG. 17-1a

FIG. 17-1b

## TECHNIQUE

1. Fold your towel so it is two inches high. Sit on towel and let ischium bones slide off the towel but not rest on the floor, causing your hips to rotate. This will aid in concaving the spine.

2. Sit tall with feet together and your belt around the balls of your feet. Clasp the belt with your left hand at about mid-thigh. Place your right wrist in back of your buttocks, as in *FIG. 17-1a.*

3. Inhale as you raise your sternum and concave your spine. Exhale while shrugging your shoulders down and back, creating a shoulder blade squeeze. Now apply the Tummy-In technique after each exhalation, and flow into the inhalation.

4. Inhale, using your finger and arm to lift your spine higher and directly onto those ischium bones. Exhale as you straighten the leg by tightening the kneecap. Pull the balls of the feet toward you so the heels raise only an inch from the floor, as in *FIG. 17-1a.*

5. Inhale, lifting up. Use your right hand and feel how your spinal column has recessed. If it has not, repeat the elongation of the spine and blade squeeze as often as is necessary to achieve the recessed spinal column. Then repeat with the other arm.

6. Only when you can do the above, should you continue. Clasp the belt now with both hands. Keep the grip at mid-thigh.

7. Do not force yourself forward and lose your concave, as in *FIG. 17-1b,* or lean back, rounding your

shoulders, as in **FIG. 17-1c.** The proper rotation of the hips, elongation of the spine, and extension and lead from the sternum will help you derive benefits from the Forward Bends. It is *not how low* you get that is important but *how well* you get there.

8. To reinforce the correct techniques, inhale again, applying the Tummy-In technique, lifting tall, and exhale while keeping sternum high. Lead forward from the hip joint, keeping your blade squeeze, as in **FIG. 17-1d.**

9. Repeat this step for 3 more rounds and as you lead with the sternum, work your elbows back, keeping them close to the body. With each inhalation, reinstate the lift from the hip. With each exhalation, increase the Forward Bend. Be aware *not* to go so far that you lose your concave.

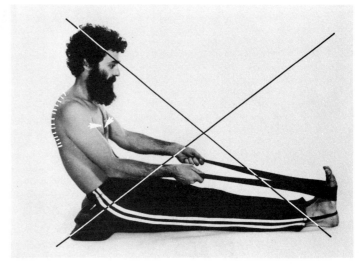

**FIG. 17-1c**

*TIPS*

1. Apply the Tummy-In technique after each exhalation to give you more room to pivot.
2. I cannot say enough for lifting and lengthening the spine. Remember, your lower back was *not* meant to sit on.
3. When the kneecap is tightened or lifted up toward the thigh, the back of the knee should be flat on the floor.
4. Make sure the belt stays under the ball of the foot and does not slide down to the arch as you are trying to flex belt forward from the ankle as in FIG. 17-d.
5. Hold at the level you can achieve, and within it relax. Take one more breath, and on the exhalation, I promise you will get further.

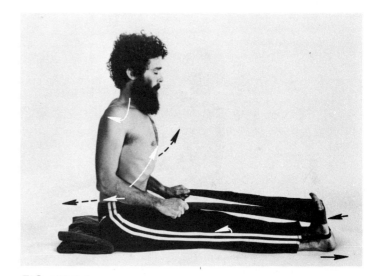

**FIG. 17-1d**

*BENEFITS*

Stretches the hamstrings.
Promotes a flexible spine.
Stimulates circulation.

### Beginner's Approach

#### TECHNIQUE

1. Sit tall and bend right leg until it is beside the right thigh and buttock. Place hands close behind you on the floor.

2. Push up on finger tips as you inhale, raising the sternum and reaching tall. Keep tall as you exhale, shrugging your shoulders back and down, away from the neck. Elbows will bend slightly.

3. Inhaling, reach tall from the hips. Exhale, concaving the back as you tighten the kneecap, and extend with the left heel, keeping the foot perpendicular to the floor, as in **FIG. 17-2a.**

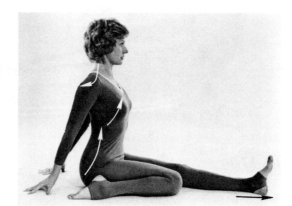

**FIG. 17-2a**

4. In this position, concentrate on taking several deep breaths in rhythm to the motions. Make sure you keep the lift on inhalation and the concaved back on exhalation. If it is a strain for you to maintain the elongation and concave, return to the previous exercise.

5. As you feel your back loosen up, you may tilt forward from the hips. Check with your hand to be sure that your back has retained the concaved position. If done correctly, the spinal column will be recessed.

6. It is extremely important that you take the time to do this exercise correctly since it is the foundation for the Forward Bends.

### Intermediate Approach

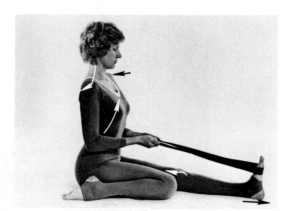

**FIG. 17-2b**

#### TECHNIQUE

**FIG. 17-2c**

1. Go from **FIG. 17-2a** to **FIG. 17-2b** by placing a belt at the ball of the left foot.

2. Inhale, extending sternum and lifting tall from the hips. As you exhale, shrug shoulders back, keeping elbows close to the body while creating a blade squeeze, as in **FIG. 17-2b.**

3. Inhaling, lift again. Exhaling, keep your knee tight and without resisting pull the foot toward the body, bending at the ankle, as in **FIG. 17-2c.**

4. Inhale as you elongate the body. Keeping the blade squeeze and back concaved, exhale completely, doing a Tummy-In and up. Now flow into another elongating inhalation. This time while exhaling,

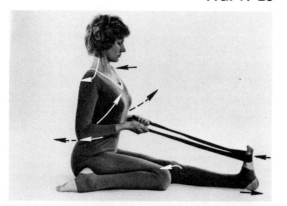

concentrate on the concaved spine, keeping elbows close to the body and working elbows towards the back. Retain the blade and squeeze, tilting forward from the hips, as in **FIG. 17-2c.**

5. Keep breathing in rhythm with the motion for 3 breaths. With each inhalation, come up part way for a good elongation. During the exhalation, draw your hands further up the belt and wing elbows out to the side as you ultimately bring your rib cage to rest on your thigh.

### Advanced Approach

*TECHNIQUE*

1. If in the preceding exercise you were able to bring your ribs to rest on your thighs, discard the belt.

2. Place right wrist on toes, cupping the ball of the foot with the fingers. Place the left hand on top of the right.

3. Holding on, inhale while you raise and extend the spine from the hips, as in **FIG. 17-2d** (left). Keep shoulders dropped, not hunched.

4. Exhaling as you lead with the sternum, squeeze the shoulder blades. Turn your hands outward to the side, bending your elbows down toward the floor, as your body follows. See **FIG. 17-2d** (right).

5. With each inhalation, raise the body just enough to give a good elongation from the hips. With each exhalation, advance down the legs.

6. Do this for 3 rounds at the lowest level you can attain without losing the concaved spine, and rest in the lower position for the count of 5. Repeat Step 5 once more and notice that you can advance even further. Now you may come up slowly and repeat on the right side.

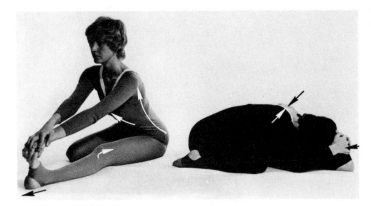

**FIG. 17-2d**

*TIPS*

1. Keep the chin raised throughout the 3 variations and lower it only if you can arrive at FIG. 17-2d (right).

2. For more details on the Tummy-In action, review Abdominal Warm-Ups. It is important to apply this technique since it gives you more room to pivot.

3. Lower your body only as far as you can without losing the recessed spine. Check with your fingers. Remember, it is not how far down you go but how well you apply the technique that counts.

4. This posture will take time to perfect. Do not jerk or force.

*BENEFITS*

Relieves tension, especially in the lumbar and shoulder areas.
Stretches and strengthens the tendons, ligaments and muscles of the legs and feet.
Limbers the spine.
Massages and firms the abdomen.

### Split Forward Bend

*TECHNIQUE*

1. Sit tall with legs approximately three feet apart. Extend the heels to straighten the legs. The outstretched foot must be vertical at all times. It is also important to keep the knee straight and kneecaps facing directly upward.

2. Place your hands on the floor directly behind you. Inhale up onto your fingertips as you elongate. Exhaling, push with the fingers, rotating the hips forward. This will bring you up directly on your ischium bones (seat bones), as in *FIG. 17-3a* (left). Place hands on left knee.

3. Inhale, extending sternum as you elongate. Exhaling, further rotate the hips to concave the spine, as in *FIG. 17-3a* (right). Lower yourself down onto the leg, using the progressive bend positions as described in "Forward Bend Pose." Repeat on the other side.

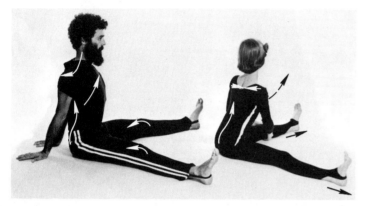

*FIG. 17-3a*

### Folded Forward Bend

*TECHNIQUE*

1. Sit with your legs stretched straight in front. Bend the left leg at the knee and move the left foot back. Place the right foot by the side of the left hip joint. Keep the toes pointing back and rest them on the floor. The inner side of the left calf will touch the outer side of the left thigh, as in *FIG. 17-3b* (left).

2. In the beginning, the body will tilt to the side of the outstretched leg. The leg and foot of the outstretched leg will also tilt outward. Learn to balance upright on your ischium bones in this position, keeping the heel extended and kneecap facing upward. When balanced you are ready to apply the techniques of the Forward Bend Pose. Then repeat, using the right leg.

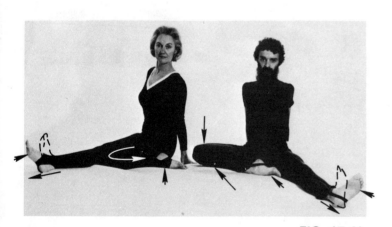

*FIG. 17-3b*

### Bent Leg Split Forward Bend

*TECHNIQUE*

1. Bend the right knee, bringing the right heel against the inner side of the right thigh near the perineum (crotch). The big toes of the right foot should touch the inner side of the left thigh, as in *FIG. 17-3b* (right). The arch of the foot should be facing directly in front of the perineum. This foot position will aid in open-

ing the leg out to the side. If this is too difficult, you can just place the right foot along the left thigh.

2. You are now in position to apply the techniques of the Forward Bend Pose of the previous exercise. Then repeat, using the left leg.

## Half-Lotus Forward Bend

### TECHNIQUE

Sit on the floor with your legs stretched in front. Bend the left leg at the knee, and place the left foot on top of the right thigh. The left heel should press the navel and the toes should be turned so the sole of the foot faces upward, as in **FIG. 17-3c** (left). Keeping the left knee on the floor, apply the techniques of the Forward Bend Pose. Then repeat on the other side.

## Bound Lotus

### TECHNIQUE

1. Repeat the Half-Lotus, as shown above, with the right foot on the left thigh.
2. Bring the right arm around the back from behind, and with an exhalation, catch the big toe of the right foot, as in **FIG. 17-3c** (right). To aid in grasping the right toe, elongate and shrug back the right shoulder. Apply the techniques of the Forward Bend Pose, then repeat on the other side.

## Bound Folded Leg

### TECHNIQUE

1. Sit with legs stretched straight. Bend the left knee and place the sole and heel of the left foot flat on the floor. The shin of the left leg should be vertical and the calf should touch the thigh. Place the left heel near the crotch. The inner side of the left foot should touch the inner side of the outstretched right thigh, as in **FIG. 17-3d** (left).
2. Stretch the left shoulder forward until the left armpit touches the vertical left shin. Turn the left arm around the left shin and thigh, bend the left elbow, and bring the left forearm behind the back at the level of the waist. Exhaling, move the right hand behind the back and clasp the left hand with the right at the wrist, as in **FIG. 17-3d** (right). If it is not possible, then clasp the palms or the fingers. Take several deep breaths in rhythm, inhaling as you elongate, and exhaling as you lower your body onto the leg.

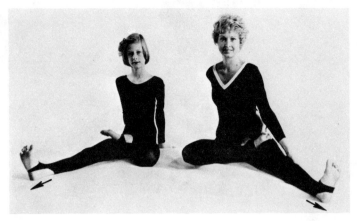

**FIG. 17-3c**

### TIPS

1. It is most important that you keep the two ischium bones even on the floor at all times.
2. Do not let the leg turn outward. The outstretched leg must be straight with heel extended, foot vertical and kneecap facing directly upward. Aligning the leg will bring you up straighter on the ischium bones. If you have difficulty keeping the leg from turning, you can place the outside of the leg along a wall.
3. If you feel a slight discomfort in the bent knee positions, make sure you first warm up your knee, using the techniques in the Lotus Warm-Ups.
4. Hold your personal level of the Forward Bend for 3 breaths, then hold, relax, and apply 1 more breath. Remember you will get further if you take time to relax.

### BENEFITS

Fully exercises the muscles of the leg.
Keeps abdominal organs healthy and firm.
Stimulates blood circulation to the spine and aids in posture.

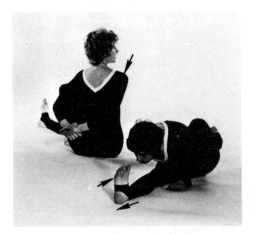

**FIG. 17-3d**

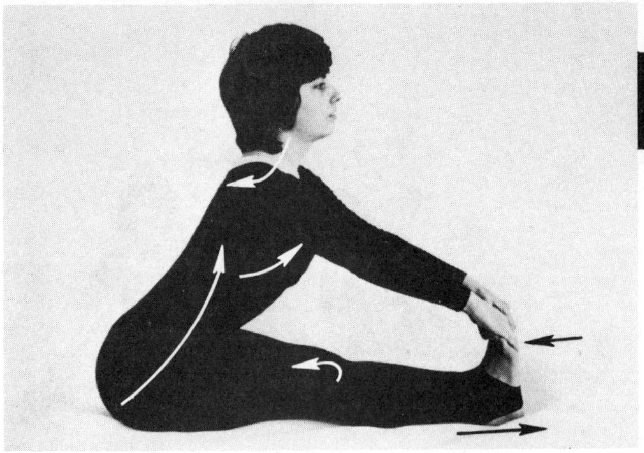

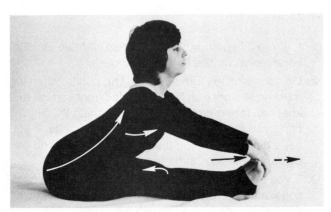

FIG. 17-4a

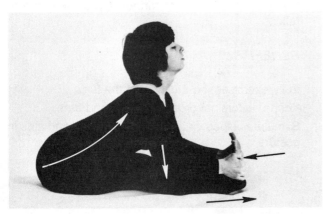

FIG. 17-4b

## ADVANCED HAND POSITIONS IN FORWARD BEND

### TECHNIQUE

1. When you have mastered the principles of the Forward Bend Pose with a good recessed spine you may proceed with this segment.
2. Sit tall with legs together in front of you, but with feet vertical. Grasp the balls of your feet with your big toes at your wrist, as in *FIG. 17-4a.*
3. Tummy-In, inhale, extend sternum, elongating the body. Exhale, concaving the spine as you continue to lower the body down to the different hand positions.
4. Push forward with the balls of your feet into hand, as in *FIG. 17-4b.* This will stretch the upper back.
5. Now, place your hand at the side of your feet, but with finger pressing so feet stay vertical. Extend yourself into the stretch by winging elbows outward as in *FIG. 17-4c.*
6. Place palms of hands together with the toe at your wrist. Continue to reach forward as far as you can go with the elbows, as in *FIG. 17-4d.* This is an extreme stretch!
7. If this is too difficult, you can grasp one of your wrists for leverage. But keep shoulders even. Come up and take a few deep breaths and relax.

### TIPS

1. While accomplishing these different hand positions, do not forget to use Tummy-In, inhale, extending sternum as you elongate, and exhale as you advance down the leg.
2. In FIG. 17-4d, cross your thumbs in order to keep hands level and shoulders even.
3. Throughout these hand positions make sure your shoulders are even to create even pressure, which will result in an equal alignment of the spine.
4. Do not rush or just pull at these stages. Your concentration point and movement is the elongation of your spine, which allows your hands to reach your personal level. Hold this level for 3 breaths, pause and relax within the position. Take 1 more complete breath and notice that you can advance even further.

### BENEFITS

Aids flexibility in the shoulders and wrist.
Good circulation of blood around abdominal organs.
It is a very invigorating pose.

FIG. 17-4c

FIG. 17-4d

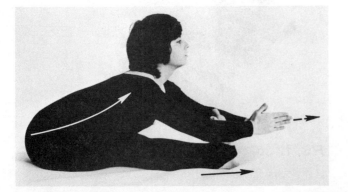

## TECHNIQUE

1. Sit tall, bending the right leg so the foot is under the left thigh. Place your hands on the thigh, inhaling as you lift up, extending the sternum, as in *FIG. 17-5a.*

2. Exhale; shrug your shoulders back and down. When exhalation is complete, pull your Tummy-In and concave the spine, reinforcing a blade squeeze. Flow into an inhalation, further elongating the body.

3. Continue Step 2, lowering your hands to grab onto feet until you have lowered your ribs onto thigh, as in *FIG. 17-5b.*

4. Come up and lean back, tipping your pelvis to help you to draw the leg up and take hold of the leg, as in *FIG. 17-5c.*

5. Looking up at the foot, inhale, extending sternum as you pull your back up straight. Exhale, shrugging shoulders back, creating a shoulder blade squeeze.

6. Completely exhale, use Tummy-In as you lift the left buttock from the floor. Inhaling, elongate higher. As you exhale, bend your elbows. Keeping the lift, bring the chest and thigh closer together. Continue breathing in rhythm with this motion for 3 breaths until you reach the position of *FIG. 17-5d.*

7. Slowly lower the left leg to the floor and repeat with the right leg.

## TIPS

1. If you have difficulty in getting a straight back in Step 5, you may place your left hand in back of your buttocks. Pushing the fingers onto the floor and straightening the arms will aid you in the lift and help you to concave the back.

2. I cannot stress enough the importance of the Tummy-In action after each exhalation. You will be using your abdominal muscles correctly, and this definitely contributes to the lift.

3. The left buttock stays off the floor throughout Step 6.

4. All through the posture the left leg is straight, with kneecaps raised toward the thigh.

## BENEFITS

Leg muscles become flexible.
Tones abdominal muscles and buttocks.
Develops balance.

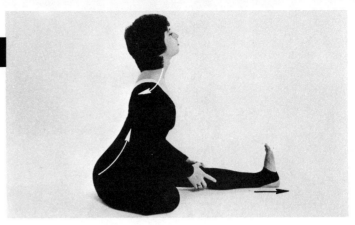

**FIG. 17-5a**

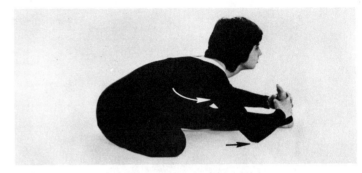

**FIG. 17-5b**

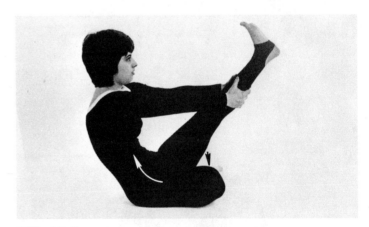

**FIG. 17-5c**

**FIG. 17-5d**

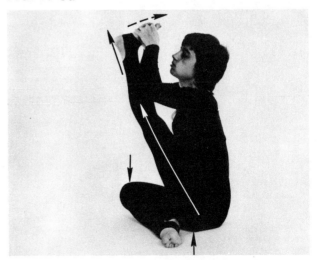

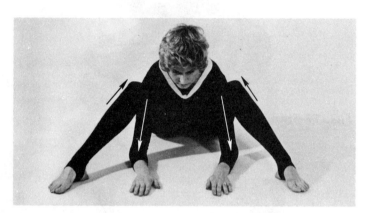

FIG. 17-6a

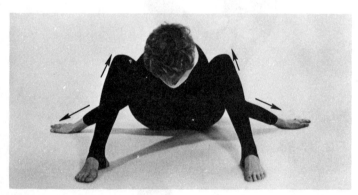

FIG. 17-6b

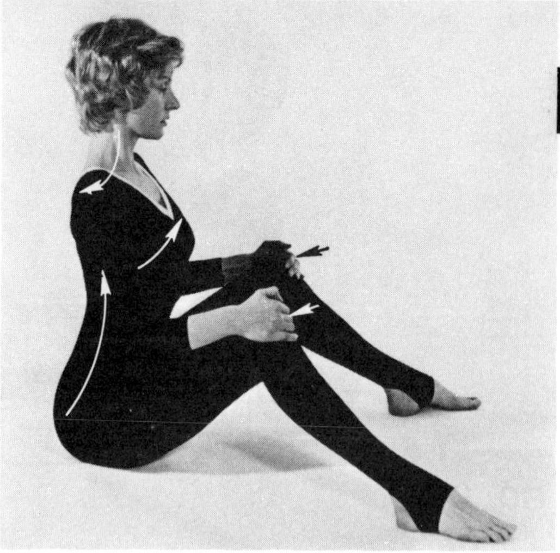

### TECHNIQUE

1. Sit on the floor with legs bent and spread wide apart, hands on your knees for leverage. Tummy-In, inhale, extend sternum as you elongate. Exhale, shrug your shoulders back and concave the spine, as in *FIG. 17-6a.*

2. Inhale, lifting up once more. Exhaling, lead from the sternum, but bend from hips as you come forward, lowering your elbows to the floor, as in *FIG. 17-6b.*

3. Once you have accomplished this, bend the knees higher so they are in line with the shoulders, as in *FIG. 17-6b.*

4. Slide your arms (elbows first) under the legs, and walk the hands beyond the buttocks and toward the back of the room. Make sure that your elbows are beyond your knees and on the outside of your thigh, as in *FIG. 17-6c.*

5. Slowly slide feet forward and hands back as you lower the head and chest to the floor, as in *FIG. 17-6d.* In this position extend your heels and feel yourself flatten to the floor. Relax! Hold for 3 breaths.

6. To come out, inch your fingers backward and your heels toward you. Then proceed to come out of it the way you went into it. Lie down and relax.

### TIPS

1. Steps 1–2 are very important in achieving this pose.
2. As for Step 3, do not go any further unless the elbows are outside of the leg.
3. Concentrate on a good exhalation as you work your head and chest toward the mat. Believe it or not, you can relax in this position.

### BENEFITS

Stretches spine and shoulder region.
Strengthens arms.
Good for circulation.

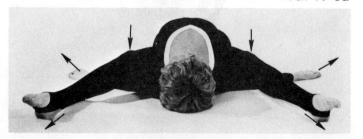

FIG. 17-6c

FIG. 17-6d

### TECHNIQUE

1. Sit tall, bend the legs outward and place one heel in front of the other, at the crotch. Lower the knees to the floor **(FIG. 17-7a)**.

2. Place the hands behind the head. You may interlock the fingers or just cup the ears.

3. Inhaling, extend sternum, lifting tall from the hips to rise straight up on your ischium bones, and concave the back **(FIG. 17-7b)**.

4. Exhaling and reaching outward to the right side, bring the right elbow to the right knee. At full exhalation, do your Tummy-In and flow into an inhalation as you elongate. Exhaling, work the left shoulder back, and do a Tummy-In. Inhaling, elongate, and this time work the right shoulder forward, bringing both arms, elbows and shoulders in line with each other **FIG. 17-7c)**.

5. At this point you are really elongating, extending the sternum, and creating a slight squeeze in the shoulders. While working the arms, you will achieve a further lift from the hips, with a good twist.

6. Keep breathing in rhythm with the motion for 3 breaths. Then repeat to the left side.

7. When you have mastered this exercise, you may lower the elbows to the floor, as in **FIG. 17-7d**, applying the same form.

8. Reaching high with raised elbow, bring yourself up to sitting position. Then, reverse to the other side.

### TIPS

1. Your knees and buttocks remain on the floor at all times.

2. As you elongate and lift up, you are working to free yourself of any wrinkles in the skin on the right side, so keep this lift within the ribs and waist as you lower to the right side. Do not slouch. If you lose the lift going down, back up and work by extending sternum and elongating to regain the lift within the pose.

3. After each exhalation, do a Tummy-In and flow into an inhalation.

4. Review Step 5.

### BENEFITS

Expands chest.
Slims waist.
Aids in doing a Lotus.

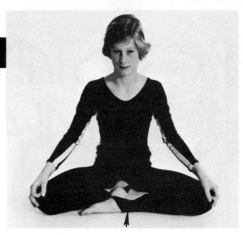

**FIG. 17-7a**

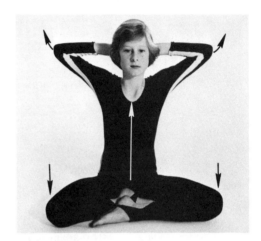

**FIG. 17-7b**

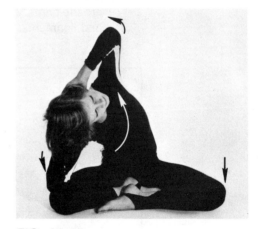

**FIG. 17-7c**
**FIG. 17-7d**

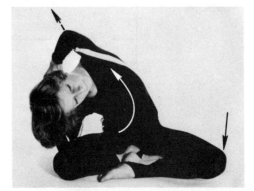

**157**

# 18 STANDING BALANCES

The ability to turn out is influenced by the strength and capacity of the muscles in the leg, in addition to the flexibility in the hip joint: the quadriceps femoris, gemellus inferior and superior, gluteus maximus and medius, and the iliacus are the primary muscles that participate in turning out, along with the hip joint and ligaments.

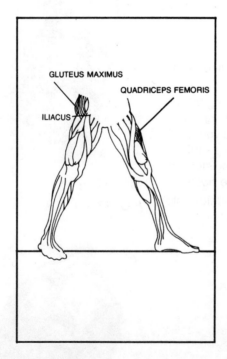

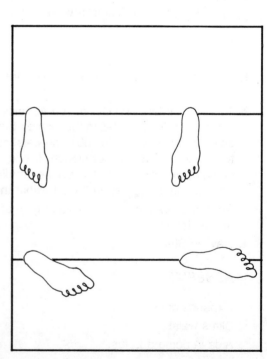

Besides strengthening these leg muscles, the following postures strengthen the abdominal muscles, by working the outward rotation in the hip joint, while keeping the rest of the body still.

I must point out that the turn out does not begin in the feet as you might have thought, but rather originates in the hip joint, ligaments and tendons that surround it. The degree of turn out depends on the student's individual pelvic construction. The ability to turn out also depends on the condition of the muscles involved in the outward leg rotation. Turn the foot out only as far as the limitation of the hip and knee joint permit, thus keeping the knee in line with the foot at all times. Tighten the knees, pull the kneecaps up, and contract the hips. The muscles in the thigh should be pulled up and rotated outward.

The turn out starts at the hip joint, passes down through the bones and muscles of the thigh to the knee joint, and finally extends to the foot.

In performing some of the following postures, you may feel you need the legs further apart. It is better to slide out the front leg while keeping the weight on the back leg, than to lose your balance and support by sliding out the back leg.

If at any time you feel tension in the lower back, it means you do not have enough pressure downward in the back leg, or you have slouched. You must maintain the continual elongation, lifting from within the hip, up the spine, and then up through the head.

These Standing Postures will develop discipline, coordination, stamina and endurance. If you just breeze through the variations, that is not correct. You must experience an inner awareness of every muscle in the body and control it to work and achieve balance for you.

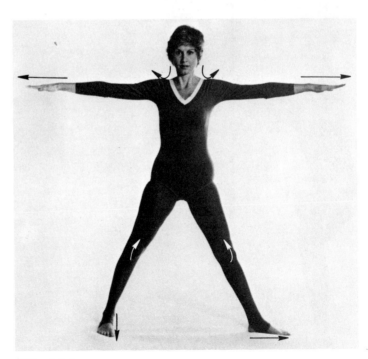

*FIG. 18-1*

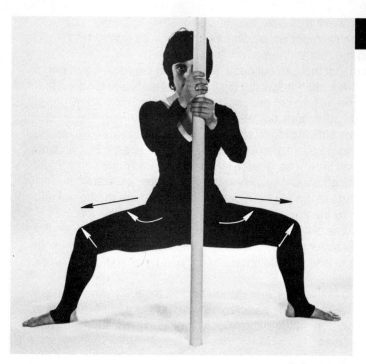

FIG. 18-2a

## TECHNIQUE

1. Find yourself an outward corner. Stand in front of it and hold onto it at arm length. Place your feet approximately 3–4 feet apart from toe to toe.

2. Inhale to elongate and align your posture, being sure to tip your pelvis. Exhale as you lower your body to "sit" without a chair, maintaining a plumb line *(FIG. 18-2a)*.

3. Your thighs should be horizontal and your shin bones should be perpendicular. If not, adjust your feet, making sure that your knees are directly over them *(FIG. 18-2b)*.

4. Hold this position for 5 breaths, working to open the thighs wider. Come up slowly to standing position.

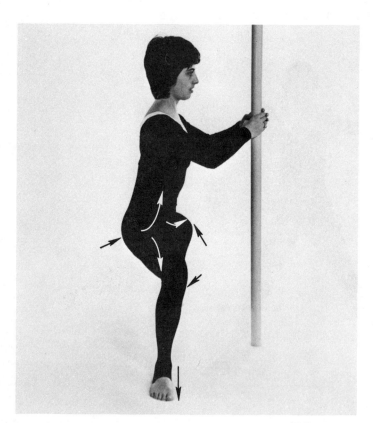

FIG. 18-2b

5. Inhale, elongating. Place your right hand on your right thigh, as in *FIG. 18-2c*. Maintain the tipped pelvis, tighten buttocks and keep back straight.

6. Keeping your plumb line, bend the right knee until it is directly over the foot, but not beyond. If the knee goes beyond the foot, slide the left foot back to make your right thigh horizontal *(FIG. 18-2d)*.

7. Be sure you keep the right knee directly over your foot as you work to keep both hips facing forward equally.

8. Hold this position for 5 breaths as you work the thigh and the hip away from each other. Slowly come up and repeat to other side. Once you achieve the correct positioning in each variation, you may move up and down or side to side to a single breath rhythm.

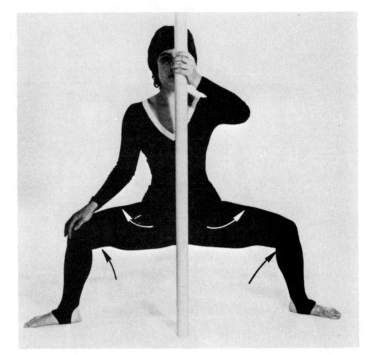

**FIG. 18-2c**

*TIPS*

**1.** If you cannot bring the knee over the toes, then bring the toes under the knee. But make sure your heel remains on the floor.

**2.** Both hips must face frontward at all times.

**3.** Keep your back straight throughout by extending sternum, making a slight blade squeeze, and tucking your tail bone under.

*BENEFITS*

Leg muscles become shapely and stronger.
Relieves cramps in calf and thigh muscles.
Tones abdominal organs.

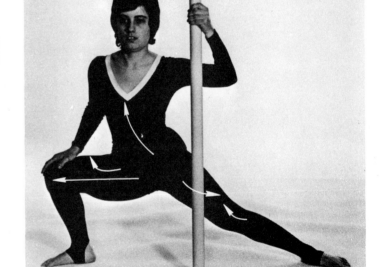

**FIG. 18-2d**

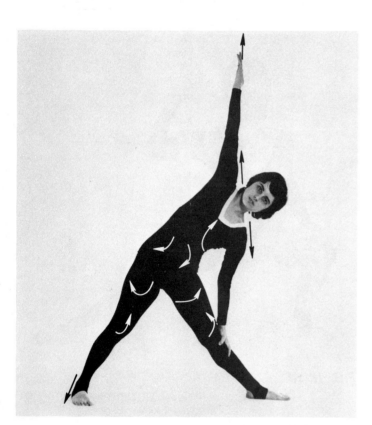

FIG. 18-3a

FIG. 18-3b

## TECHNIQUE

1. Stand and spread legs three feet apart. Rotate the entire leg, pivoting on the heel as you turn left foot out to side at a right angle. Rotate and pivot the right leg and foot inward 3 inches. Now rotate the thighs outward as arrows indicate. This will aid in keeping your hips forward. Raise the arms out sideways in line with the shoulders, palms facing down and reaching outward to open shoulder blades. Tighten the legs by raising kneecaps.

2. Inhale, lifting your ribs upward. Exhale as you lead with the left arm out, followed by the extended (left) ribs, as in **FIG. 18-3a,** lowering the trunk until the left hand meets the leg **(FIG. 18-3b).**

3. Inhale as you extend your right arm higher, from the shoulder blade. Check to make sure your kneecaps and buttocks are tight to help keep the right hip from moving. If the hips still will not stay aligned, turn your right thigh outward by shifting more weight to the outside of the right foot.

4. Exhale, apply the Tummy-In technique, then continue in this position for 3 breaths. (Exhale, Tummy-In, extend the spine; inhale; exhale further, twisting to align over the left leg.)

5. If you still find it difficult please do not go on. It is important to perfect the basic positioning before going on. To aid in your position balance and alignment, place yourself against a wall and continue from Step 1.

6. To help achieve position: make sure the back of the legs, back of the chest, and hips are in line. Look at the thumb of the outstretched right hand. Keep the left knee raised and in line with the toes. Bring the left shoulder and hip forward to get the correct alignment.

7. Inhale as you elongate the trunk, and exhale while continuing to stretch into this posture, bringing your left hand further down the leg, with the ultimate goal being the ankle, without turning the hip. If you bend yourself at the half-way mark, it is helpful to place your hand on a box or books *(FIG. 18-3c)*.

8. Limber folks should rest the left palm flat on the floor either at the outside of the left foot or on the inside of the left foot *(FIG. 18-3d)*. Turn from the ear to bring the chin in line with the shoulder as you look toward the outstretched right hand.

9. Remain in this position taking 3 deep and even breaths. Then lifting up with the right arm, bring yourself up. Repeat to the other side.

### TIPS

1. To help you accomplish the preliminary alignment for this posture, do it with your back against the wall, heels three inches out from the wall. This will remind you to tip your pelvis, keep your buttocks tight, with hip facing forward and shoulder over your leg.

2. Again, I stress the importance of working to rotate the hip open to bring it forward.

3. To help, use your right hand on the right hip to turn and open it outward.

4. In Step 8, if there is any tension in the neck, keep head facing toward, as in FIG. 18-3c.

5. Make sure you do not lose the supported balance in the right hip, down the tightened leg to the heel and outer edge of the right foot. The back leg is the anchor of all the following Standing Balances.

### BENEFITS

Tones hip, thigh and leg muscles.
Relieves menstrual cramps.
Strengthens ankles.

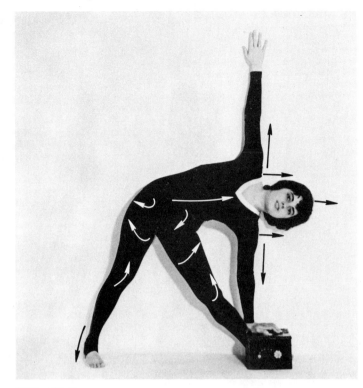

**FIG. 18-3c**

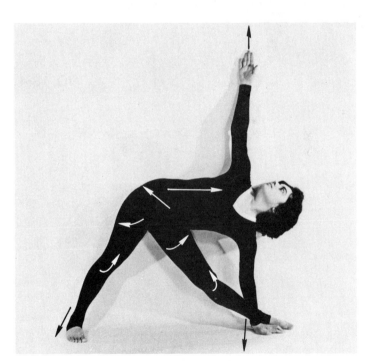

**FIG. 18-3d**

163

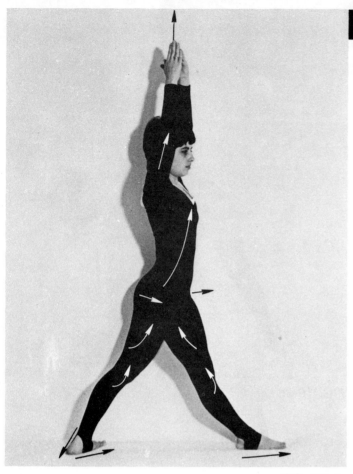

**FIG. 18-4a**

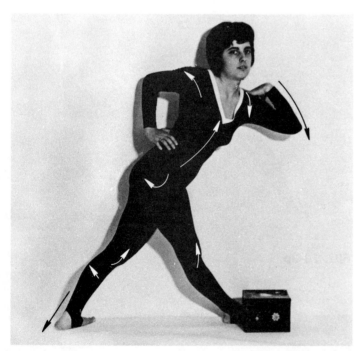

**FIG. 18-4b**

## TECHNIQUE

1. Stand facing the wall with feet three feet apart. Raise your arms over head. Rotate the leg, pivoting on the heel as you turn the right foot out. Rotate and pivot the left leg and foot inward slightly, keeping the hips forward.

2. Inhale as you lift tall, and exhale as you rotate the trunk and hips until directly facing the right (see **FIG. 18-4a**). Check to see if you have your sternum in line with your knee and foot. Make sure the support of your foot comes from the ball and heel first, then from the outer edge, of the left foot. Maintain support under the big toe of the right foot. Make sure you have tightened the legs by raising the kneecaps. Also squeeze the upper thighs together for balance.

3. Inhale as you lead with your left elbow (see **FIG. 18-4b**). Exhale as you begin to extend outward, and lower the body. Continue to take even elongating breaths as you twist, aligning your elbow with the

outside of the right foot. When you are low enough, lower the palm on the box (see *FIG. 18-4c*), or palm down on the outside of the right foot (see *FIG. 18-4d*).

4. Stretch the right arm up, bringing it in line with left arm (see *FIG. 18-4c*). Look up at your right hand.

5. When you are in this position, bring left shoulder forward and right shoulder back with shoulder blade pulled down.

6. In this position, take only 3 breaths as you stretch horizontally further into the move, rotating the left side of the body toward the right, applying the Tummy-In technique after each exhalation to elongate further.

7. Inhale as you lift and reach with the right arm, rotate the trunk back to its original position and come back to *FIG. 18-4a*.

8. Exhale, repeat the pose on the left side by turning the left foot out and right foot in (reversing the position).

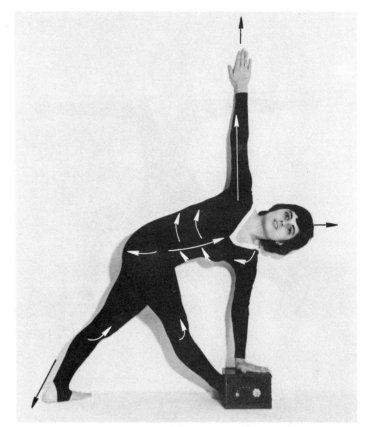

**FIG. 18-4c**

### TIPS

1. If you are having difficulty with your balance in the middle of the room, you may adapt this posture by using a wall (as pictured).

2. Be careful not to lose the supported balance in the left hip, down the tightened leg to the heel. This is the anchor of the pose.

3. It is helpful to bring the left shoulder forward and the right shoulder back, so arms, shoulders, and head are against the wall.

4. In the Triangle Twist, *balance* is the aim. As I have said previously, it is not important how far down you get in these exercises; if you lose your balance and inner awareness, you have accomplished nothing.

### BENEFITS

Tones thigh, calf and hamstring muscles.
Invigorates the abdominal organs.
Strengthens hip muscles.

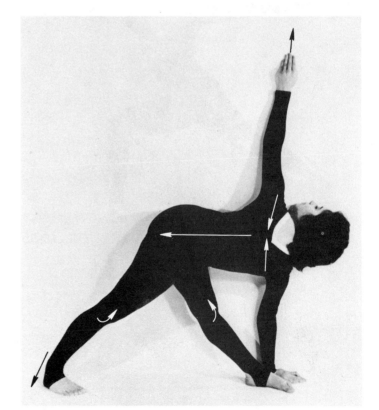

**FIG. 18-4d**

## LATERAL ANGLE POSE

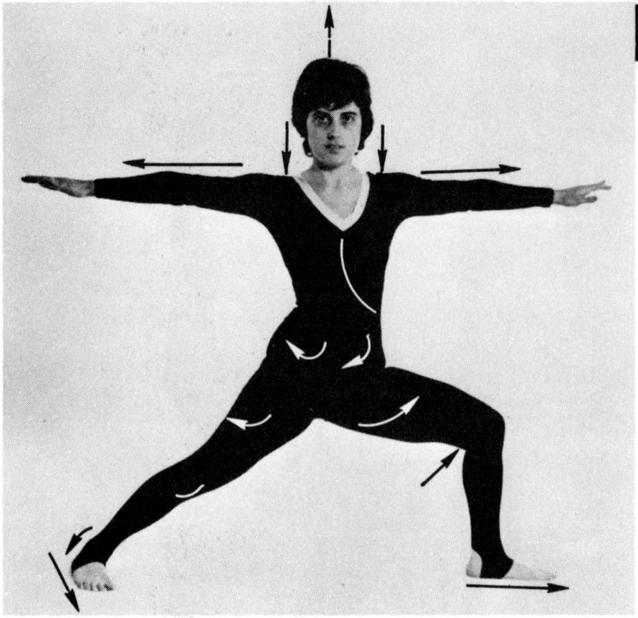

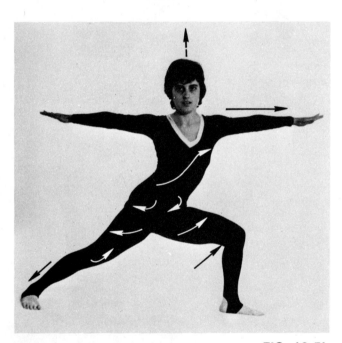

FIG. 18-5a

FIG. 18-5b

### TECHNIQUE

1. Stand with legs four feet apart. Raise arms in line with shoulders. Pivot on the heel, turning the left foot out and the right foot in. Keep hips facing forward by tipping pelvis, tightening buttocks and kneecaps.
2. Inhale as you lift your trunk up while keeping shoulders down.
3. Exhale, leading with the left side of your rib cage and left arm, maintaining a straight plumb line as you lower, and bending the left knee until the thigh and calf form a right angle and the left thigh is parallel to the floor ***(FIG. 18-5a).*** Keep the right leg straight and the kneecap raised as the weight presses to the outer edge of the right foot.
4. Inhaling, stretch tall; extend your sternum. Exhale, extending the left side of your rib cage and the left arm further to the side ***(FIG. 18-5b).***

5. Inhale as you elongate the trunk diagonally. Exhale as you continue to stretch out and down. Place left palm on the floor, by the side of the left foot; the left armpit is covering and touching the outer side of the left knee *(FIG. 18-5c)*.

6. While in this position, you are concentrating on using your right hand to turn your right hip up. Tighten the right leg and keep the support on the outer edge of the right foot. The chest, hips, and legs should be in a line; and in order to achieve this, move the chest up and twist back, extending the spine from the face toward the head.

7. Stretch the right arm upward and out over the right ear. Keep your head in line with the spine *(FIG. 18-5d)*.

8. Stretch every part of the body, especially the spine, until all the vertebrae and ribs move and you feel a sensation that the skin is being stretched and pulled.

9. In this position take 3 good elongating breaths, applying the Tummy-In technique. To come up, inhale, reaching the right arm and shoulder up high, and lift yourself up. Exhale as you straighten out your left leg; return to standing position. Repeat to the right side.

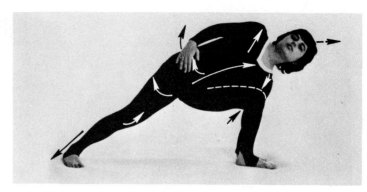

**FIG. 18-5c**

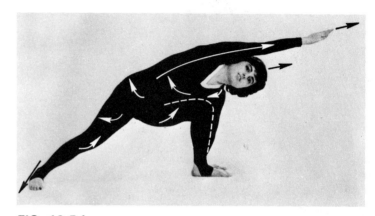

**FIG. 18-5d**

## TIPS

1. Throughout the above moves, make sure the bent knee is directly in line with the foot. Otherwise you are risking straining your knee.

2. In FIG. 18-5c, the knee and arm are constantly challenging each other.

3. Believe it or not, the left baby finger pressing onto the floor has a lot to do with balance.

4. Remember, to aid in the twist of the rib cage, take your hand and pull yourself around.

## BENEFITS

Tones up ankles, knees and thighs.
Reduces waist and hips.
Relieves sciatic and arthritic pain.

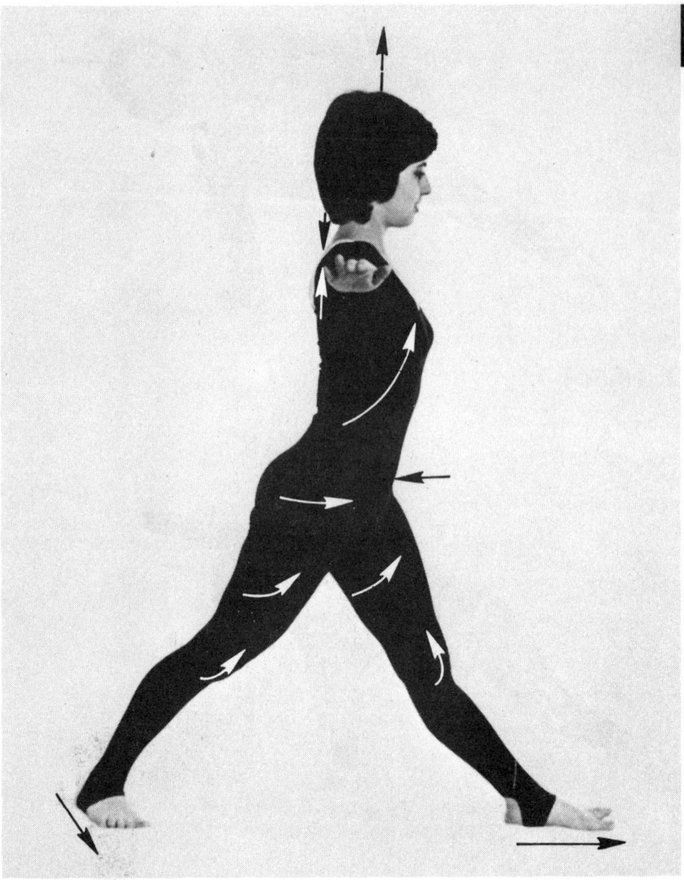

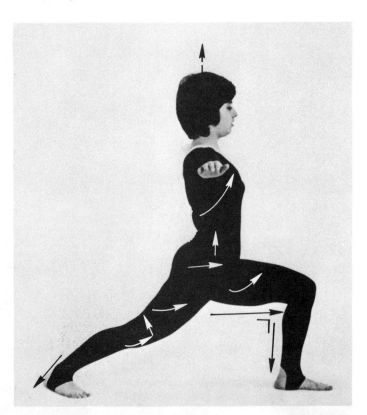

FIG. 18-6a

### TECHNIQUE

1. Stand with arms at shoulder level, with legs four feet apart.

2. Inhale as you lift up from the waist.

3. Exhale as you rotate the legs and pivot on the left heel, turning the foot out. Rotate and pivot, turning the right foot in slightly. Make sure legs are straight with kneecaps up.

4. Inhale, once more lifting up from the waist. Exhale as you rotate from the hips to face the left foot, squeezing the upper thighs together. Make sure the right hip is even with your left hip; if not, move right hip forward *(FIG. 18-6a)*.

5. Exhale, as you bend the left knee until the left thigh is parallel to floor and the left shin perpendicular to floor, forming a right angle between the left thigh and left calf. The bent knee should not extend beyond the ankle but should be in line with the heel *(FIG. 18-6b)*.

FIG. 18-6b

6. Inhale as you raise your arms, stretching up over-head. Lift from your ribs, not your shoulders. The neck remains centered and relaxed with elbows locked and arms up by the ears *(FIG. 18-6c)*.

7. Make sure your right leg is straight and you are still tight at the knee, focusing the weight on the outer edge of the back foot. If you feel pressure in the lower back, you have sagged. Tip your pelvis and lift up high from the hips. This is important.

8. Inhale, and lift up, exhaling with arched back, and keeping ears in line with arms. Even in this position, there should not be any pressure in the lower back *(FIG. 18-6d)*. If so, elongate the spine.

9. Maintain this pose for 2–3 breaths. Apply the Tummy-In action to further elongate. Come out of it the same way as you went into it, and repeat on the other side.

## TIPS

1. Make sure your bent knee is directly over your heel. If not, you are putting excess pressure on your knee.
2. If you cannot keep the back heel on the floor, do this posture with the heel against a wall. It will help you balance.
3. This exercise is particularly strenuous. It should neither be tried by persons with weak hearts, nor held for too long by anyone.

## BENEFITS

Relieves stiffness in shoulders and back.
Tones up ankles and knees.
Reduces fat around the hips.

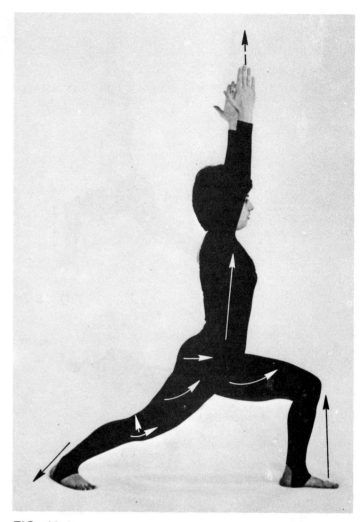

**FIG. 18-6c**

**FIG. 18-6d**

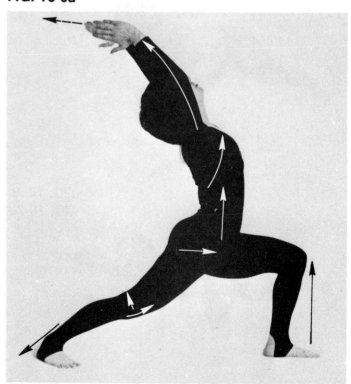

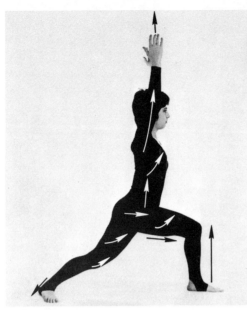

FIG. 18-7a

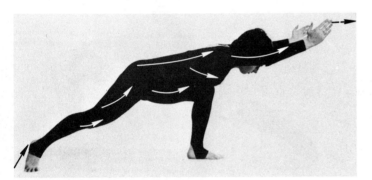

FIG. 18-7b

FIG. 18-7c
FIG. 18-7d

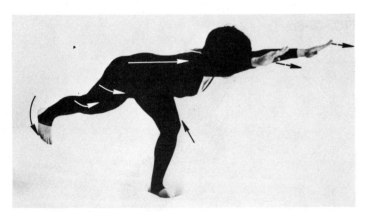

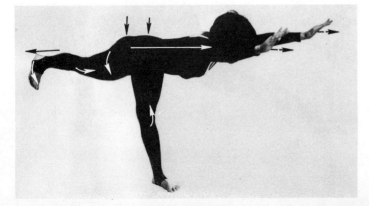

## TECHNIQUE

1. This posture is an intensified continuation of the Standing Plunge.
2. Stand with legs four feet apart. Work to the final pose of the Standing Plunge on the left side *(FIG. 18-7a)*.
3. Inhale as you stretch up from the hips. Exhale and reach forward into bending posture, and place the chest on the left thigh *(FIG. 18-7b)*. Do not slouch. Keep that reach in the straight arms.
4. Inhale, reaching forward even more. As you exhale, extend your trunk toward the hands, raising the back leg while straightening the left leg *(FIG. 18-7c)*. Then completely straighten the left leg *(FIG. 18-7d)*. Remember to raise your kneecap.
5. Maintain this position for 3 breaths as you do the next movement.
6. As you balance, keep the whole body (except for the left leg) parallel to the floor. The left leg is to be fully stretched and kept perpendicular to the floor. Pull back of your right thigh while stretching your arms and right leg, as if two persons were pulling you from either end. Do not point toe, but extend heel. All this is worked on during your 3 breaths.
7. Exhale down slowly the same way you went into the "T" Pose, and return to the original standing position.
8. Repeat on the right side.

### TIPS

1. When you are in the position of FIG. 18-7b, you may turn your right foot around so it is facing in the same direction as the left foot. This will help you in your lift.
2. In FIG. 18-7d your buttocks should be level. If not, turn your right foot inward. This will lower your right buttock.
3. I cannot stress enough the importance of the continual stretch throughout the Pose in order to achieve balance and its benefits.

### BENEFITS

Contracts and tones abdominal organs.
Relieves cramps in calf and thigh muscles.
Brings elasticity to leg and back muscles.

170

## TECHNIQUE

1. Place your palms together between shoulder blades (see **FIG. 18-8a**). Stand with feet 3½–4 feet apart. Rotate the leg and pivot on your left heel to turn the foot to the side. Rotate and pivot the right foot in (see **FIG. 18-8b**).

2. Inhale, raising your chest and ribs. Keep shoulders and neck relaxed.

3. Exhale as you turn your trunk and hips to the side, directly in line with the left foot, squeezing the upper thighs together. Make sure the hip bones are even and the sternum lines up with the left foot.

4. Inhale as you lift your trunk, expanding your chest to make breathing easier, and extend your chin up (see **FIG. 18-8b**). Remember the anchor of the pose is in the back right hip, knee, and foot.

5. Keeping the knees tight throughout, exhale as you bend forward, lowering and leading your body from the sternum **(FIG. 18-8c)**. Apply the Tummy-In technique and inhale as you elongate. Then exhaling slowly, lower the chest onto the left leg **(FIG. 18-8d)**. Hold for a slow count of 5 with normal breathing, further elongate so that your hip and rib touch the thigh and your chin moves down the shin.

6. To come up, inhale as you arch your head up, shoulders and elbows back, concaving the spine. Keep feet firmly onto the floor. Then exhale (as illustrated in **FIG. 18-8c**); then go to **FIG. 18-8b** position.

7. You are now through with one side. Do not give up; reverse the feet position and repeat. You can rest afterward.

## TIPS

1. It is very important that you keep both hips turned directly to the side, facing the extended foot.
2. Concentrate on your foot position as well as on how you are using your feet. The toes are relaxed, but you press the ball of the foot onto the floor. This along with the pressure you apply with the heels and outer edge of your back foot is also very important for maintaining balance.

## BENEFITS

Relieves stiffness in leg and hip muscles.
Makes the hip joints and spine more elastic.
Corrects round and droopy shoulders.

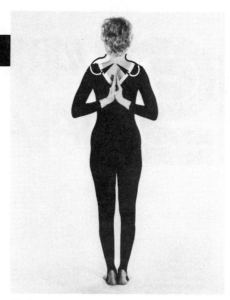

FIG. 18-8a

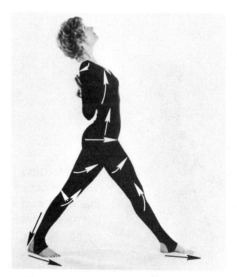

FIG. 18-8b

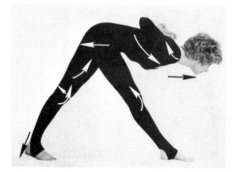

FIG. 18-8c
FIG. 18-8d

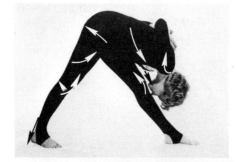

# 19 VARIED BALANCES

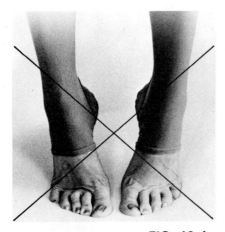

**FIG. 19-1a**

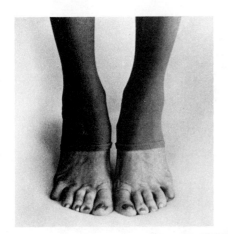

**FIG. 19-1b**

I want to discuss again here where one's balance begins—the feet.

Almost all of us are born with perfect feet. It is the abuse we give them that makes us limp into adulthood. The foot is delicately balanced and one of the most complicated joints in the body. We have injured and insulted our feet by squeezing them into shoes of various styles (high heels, heavy shoes, sloped heels and platforms), thereby causing either tension or locked joints, strain in the muscles, limitation of foot motion, or a combination of all of these disturbances. Feet that roll out or in may have been caused by badly outworn shoes and these foot conditions are responsible for sprained ankles, fallen arches, etc.

Most foot disabilities result from poor posture in standing and walking. The student who suffers from foot strain can best acquire relief by learning how to stand correctly and doing special exercises to strengthen weak and stretched foot muscles.

In executing most postures, the student must align the knee directly over the properly placed foot. A knee that is not properly positioned is very vulnerable to excessive strain in the knee joint.

As you do the following postures, concentrate on the positioning of the feet. The weight should be equally distributed between the ball and heel, with toes relaxed. In preparation for the Squatting Balances, go up on your toes. If your feet look like **FIG. 19-1a,** you are wrong. Bring your ankle in to realign your feet and legs, as in **FIG. 19-1b.** Come down slowly and relax. The first two postures which follow in this chapter concentrate on balancing equally on both ischium bones.

To aid you in the following balancing postures, it will help greatly if you will fix your gaze on a spot on the floor, your height's distance away, as in **DIAGRAM 1.** (Your height's distance will depend on the degree of height you have at the start of a given posture, as in **DIAGRAMS 2** and **3.)** Observing this "Range of Vision" will help you keep your balance, giving imaginary support

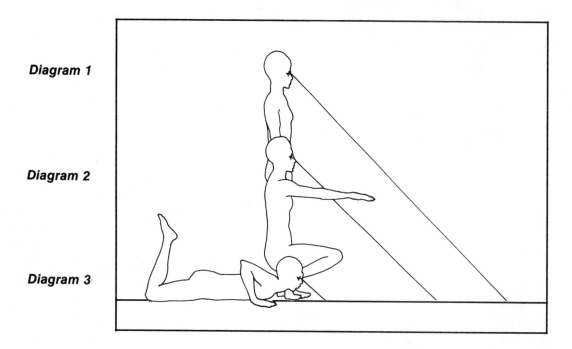

**Diagram 1**

**Diagram 2**

**Diagram 3**

from the eyes to "your" spot and a sense of stability to the body.

Breathe evenly throughout these postures. This will aid in bringing smoothness and coordinated action during the postures. The student uses his ocular reflexes to the maximum.

An understanding of anatomy and a mental placement of your body enables you to develop correctly and efficiently.

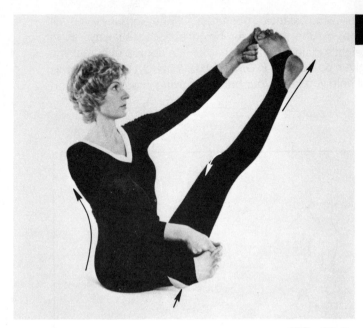

FIG. 19-2a

### Split

#### TECHNIQUE

1. Sit tall, bending your legs so the soles of the feet are together. Wrap the index fingers around the inside of the big toes. Place your thumb on top of the nail.

2. Inhale, extend sternum, and elongate, concaving the spine, and sitting centered on the ischium bones. Exhaling, tilt back, working to maintain the concaved spine as you raise the feet slightly from the floor.

3. Inhale, lift up, extend sternum, creating a shoulder blade squeeze. Exhale as you keep the lift, and straighten the left leg out to the side *(FIG. 19-2a)*.

4. To achieve balance, incorporate the above pointer as you continue to inhale (lifting up). Exhale, raising the right leg up straight *(FIG. 19-2b)*.

5. With each completed exhalation, do the Tummy-In and up as you elongate, and inhale.

6. Take 3 deep breaths within this position to maintain the proper balance. When this is achieved, bring the legs together. Then lower the legs and relax.

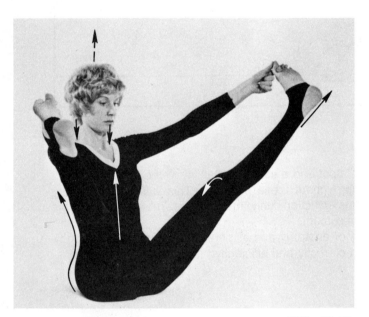

FIG. 19-2b

### TECHNIQUE

1. Sit tall on your ischium bones. Holding onto the legs, bring them close to the chest. The feet are off the floor *(FIG. 19-2c)*.
2. Exhale completely, do your Tummy-In and up, and flow into an inhalation elongating. Create a shoulder blade squeeze.
3. When you find your balance point, maintain the lift as you straighten out your leg, placing the arms at shoulder level *(FIG. 19-2d)*.
4. Hold this position for 3 breaths. Slowly come down and enjoy the feeling of accomplishment.

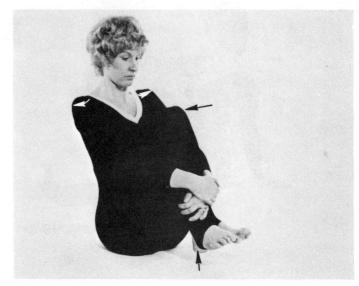

**FIG. 19-2c**

### TIPS

1. You may attempt Step 3, FIG. 19-2a with the foot on the floor to work toward the proper lift. When this is accomplished, raise the foot as shown.
2. Do not let your back sag. You will roll over backward.
3. The shoulder blade squeeze and lift is the secret to this balance.

### BENEFITS

Tones waist and inner thighs.
Strengthens the spine.
Stimulates abdominal muscles.

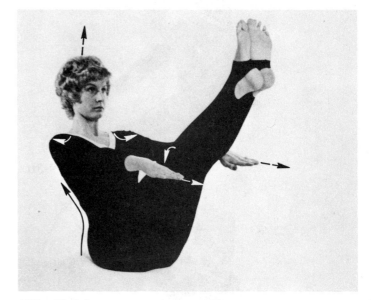

**FIG. 19-2d**

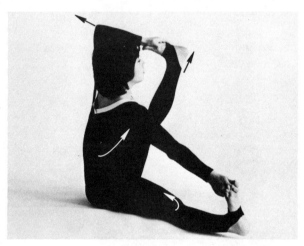

**FIG. 19-3a**

## TECHNIQUE

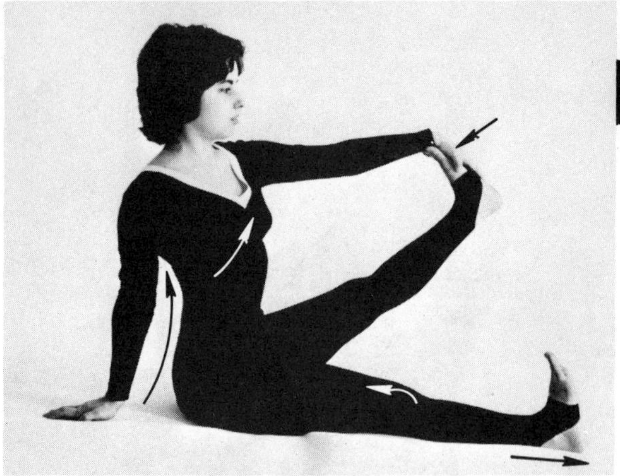

1. Sit up tall with legs stretched straight out in front. Bend the left knee, and grab hold of the foot with your left hand. Exhale as you straighten out the left leg *(FIG. 19-3a)*. If you can do this, you should be able to accomplish the following. So lower the leg and begin.

2. Wrap the index fingers around the inside of the big toes. Place the thumb on top of the toe nail.

3. Bend the left leg. Inhale, elongating, while you tilt directly onto the right buttock and leg. The left buttock is completely off the floor.

4. Keeping the elongation, exhale as you straighten the left leg *(FIG. 19-3b)*. Take 3 breaths (inhaling, keeping the lift; exhaling, straightening the back) as you work to a steady balance.

5. As you acquire the necessary lift, bend the left elbow to the shin bone *(FIG. 19-3c)*. Take 3 breaths in this position. Then repeat to the other side.

6. Now that you are warmed up, bend the left knee, exhale and pull the left foot up until the heel is close to the ear. At the same time, draw the left arm back from the shoulder *(FIG. 19-3d)*. Take 3 breaths, reviewing Step 4. Slowly come down and repeat to the other side.

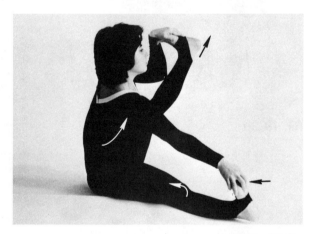

**FIG. 19-3b**

**FIG. 19-3c**

**FIG. 19-3d**

## TIPS

1. Do not let go of the right big toe. Work to keep the right heel extended, kneecap raised and entire leg resting on the floor.

2. Also keep the raised leg absolutely straight.

3. The above pointers are correct, but if you cannot reach the right toe, hold on to where you *can* reach.

4. During the final stage of each posture apply a Tummy-In action.

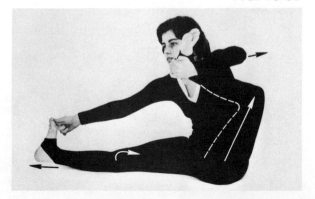

## BENEFITS

Stimulates abdominal muscles, spine and neck. Keeps muscles of legs and thighs elastic and strong. Stretches hamstring muscles and makes hip joints flexible.

## TECHNIQUE

1. Assume perfect posture position with feet apart at hip-distance. Exhale as you rise straight up on your toes. Check ankle position.
2. Elongate as you inhale raising your arms out front to shoulder level *(FIG. 19-4a)*.
3. To lower, exhale, tightening your buttocks and keeping your back straight *(FIG. 19-4b)*. Do not lean forward. Slowly lower the body to squatting position *(FIG. 19-4c)*.
4. Inhale, reaching forward for counter-balance. Exhaling, lower your heels to the floor *(FIG. 19-4d)*.
5. Inhale, roll back onto the toes. Exhale, retracting your arms to realign shoulders *(FIG. 19-4c)*.
6. Inhale, elongating as you raise your arms overhead, and clasp your hands. Exhaling, slowly raise your body straight up without leaning forward. You may now come down onto your heels and relax.

## TIPS

1. Keep your ankles in with weight evenly distributed on the balls of your feet without gripping toes.
2. If you have difficulty lowering your heels to the floor, place feet further apart.
3. Keep eyes on your range of vision throughout this exercise.
4. To come up or down you must keep your back elongated, straight, and vertical, with your shoulders back and relaxed.

## BENEFITS

Strengthens legs and ankles.
Exercises thigh muscles.
Corrects minor leg problems.

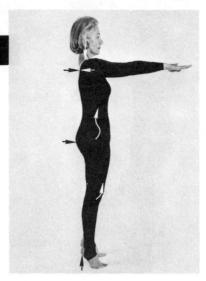

FIG. 19-4a

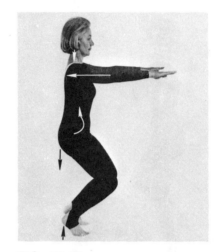

FIG. 19-4b

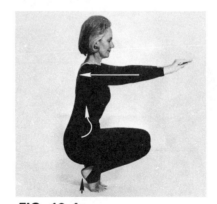

FIG. 19-4c

FIG. 19-4d

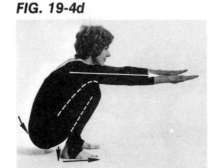

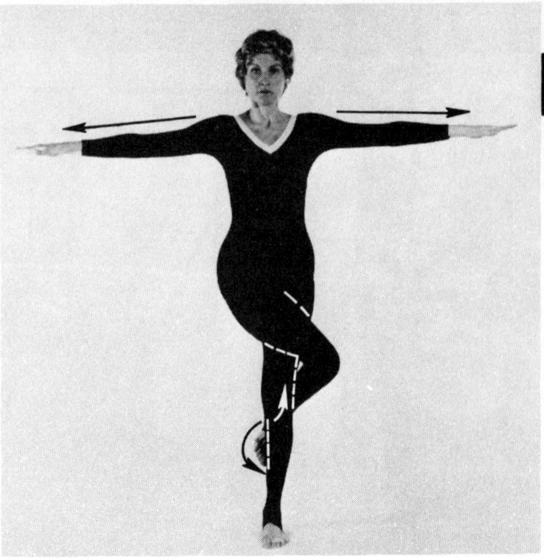

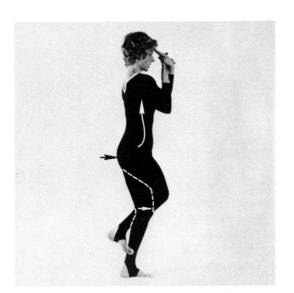

FIG. 19-5a

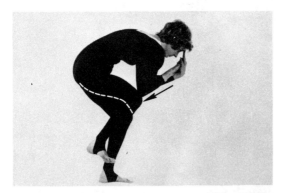

FIG. 19-5b

## EAGLE POSE

### TECHNIQUE

1. Stand straight. Swing your right leg around the front of the supporting left leg, wrapping your right ankle around the lower left leg until your right toes point to the front just above the inner side of the left ankle *(FIG. 19-5a)*. While in this position, inhale as you elongate, and exhale as you intertwine your arms and balance with your finger on the forehead *(FIG. 19-5b)*.

2. When you can maintain this balance easily, inhale, then exhale as you lower elbows onto the knee *(FIG. 19-5c)*. Now extend the elbows outward and bend forward until your chin and sternum rest on your bent upper leg so that your entire body is folded inward *(FIG. 19-5d)*. Hold for the count of 5.

3. Slowly come up with the same control as you went down. Repeat with other leg.

### TIPS

1. Check your range of vision to help in keeping balance.
2. In all of these balancing postures, one should come out of them as slowly and gracefully as one went into them.

### BENEFITS

Creates poise and grace.
Reduces waistline.
Tones leg muscles.

FIG. 19-5c

FIG. 19-5d

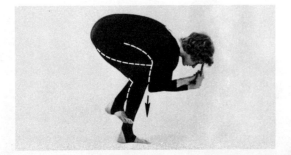

### TECHNIQUE

1. Stand up straight. Bend the right knee, taking the right foot in both hands. With the knee turned out to the side in a Half-Lotus position, work the foot as high up the front of the left leg as you can. Secure your foot by having the left kneecap raised, the ball of the foot firmly on the floor, and your ankle aligned with the foot. Inhale and raise both hands over your head *(FIG. 19-6a)*.

2. Exhale, bend from the hips, lower your back as you slowly lower your hands, touching down onto your finger tips about 1 foot in front of your toes *(FIG. 19-6b)*.

3. Inhale once more to elongate, then exhale as you bring the palms by the side of the feet *(FIG. 19-6c)*. Turn palms toward the back *(FIG. 19-6d)*.

4. Inhale as you come up slowly, still keeping your balance on one leg with kneecap up. Raise your arms over head and exhale as you lower them to the sides, slowly placing the foot back on the floor.

5. Take a few deep breaths, then repeat with other leg.

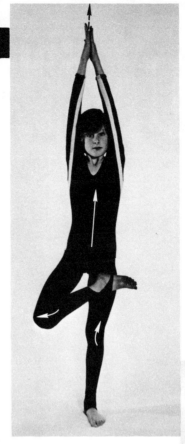

**FIG. 19-6a**

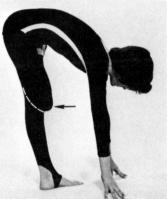

**FIG. 19-6b**

### TIPS

1. Check your range of vision to help in your balance.
2. It is important to get the foot high enough into the groin so that you can bend properly.
3. It is most important that you keep the bent knee out to the side as you lower, so do not place incorrect pressure on the knee.
4. It is helpful to apply pressure with your right foot against the left upper leg, to aid in working that knee out to the side.
5. In Step 2 apply the Tummy-In action.

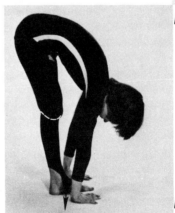

**FIG. 19-6c**

**FIG. 19-6d**

### BENEFITS

Develops flexibility in hips.
Increases suppleness in the spine.
Aids in coordination and balance.

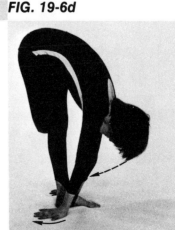

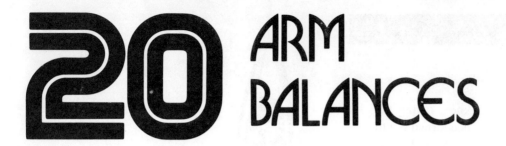

# 20 ARM BALANCES

The usefulness and flexibility of the hand depends on the variety of positions made possible by the elbow, forearm and shoulder joints.

The forearm is made up of two long bones, the ulna and the radius, which meet with the humerus, the long bone of the upper arm. The rotational movement of the forearm occurs at the articulation between the radius and ulna, not at the elbow joint.

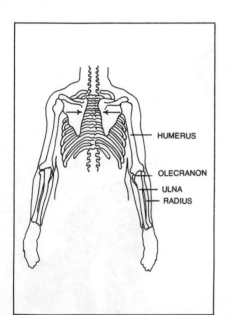

HUMERUS

OLECRANON
ULNA
RADIUS

INCORRECT

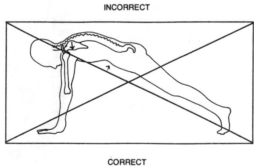

CORRECT

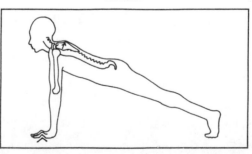

Hyperextended elbow joints are caused by a short olecranon (a part of the ulna that forms the point of the elbow) process, rather than a loose ligament in the joint. Girls are prone to this irregularity because of the female skeleton pattern. To improve or disguise this, just keep the elbow rounded and up, avoiding full extension of the arm.

Before you go into the balancing exercises, it will help greatly to learn proper hand positioning.

Do not grip your fingertips into the mat so much that the palms of the hands lift from the floor. The correct way is to spread your fingers wide and concave both first knuckles nearest the nail; this places the pads of your fingers firmly onto the floor. Your second knuckles are bent upward, forming an inverted "V" with the last third of the fingers, thereby pressing the whole palm of the hand onto the floor. This gives you added strength and a proper foundation for the base of your balancing postures.

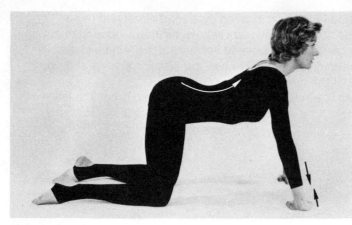

**FIG. 20-1a**

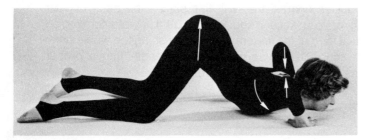

**FIG. 20-1b**

## Chin And Chest Push-Up

*TECHNIQUE*

1. Lie face down with your legs hip-distance apart with fingers pointing to the chest, just below the shoulders. Push your hands onto the floor to bring you up into a kneeling position *(FIG. 20-1a)*. Do not move your toes or hands, and keep your chin up.

2. Inhale, extending sternum. Keep buttocks high. Exhale, slowly lowering your chest and chin to the floor while creating a tight shoulder blade squeeze *(FIG. 20-1b)*.

3. Inhale, pausing here a moment to check that shoulders are not hunched up at the ears. Shoulders are away from the ears, but maintaining blade squeeze.

4. Exhale as you push up until your arms are completely straight.

5. Repeat the above until you have accomplished the coordination of the blade squeeze without hunching the shoulders up at the ears.

6. To advance, inhale, extending and leading from the sternum as you lower to the floor. Exhale as you push yourself up, keeping the shoulder blade squeeze. Repeat 4 times.

## Kneeling Push-Up

### TECHNIQUE

1. Assume the position of Step 1, but place feet up toward the ceiling and hands facing forward. With face down, tighten buttocks, then put the palms of your hands onto the floor as you raise yourself up into a perfectly straight incline *(FIG. 20-1c).*

2. Inhale; extend sternum and lead with it as you lower yourself (parallel to the floor) see *FIG. 20-1d.* Do not hunch, and keep blade squeeze.

3. Exhaling, keep your blade squeeze, as you push yourself up until you are in a straight incline.

4. Repeat the above as often as you wish, but stop if you lose your alignment.

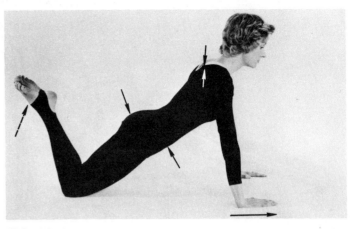

**FIG. 20-1c**

### TIPS

1. To come up, it is helpful to press the heel of your hand onto the floor.
2. Keep the feet up. This will aid in keeping buttocks tight and spine in alignment.
3. Tip pelvis slightly to keep your abdomen in.
4. Keep neck relaxed; do not thrust it forward.

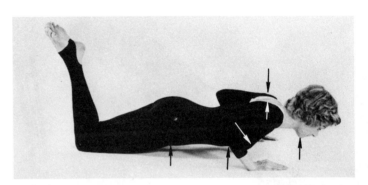

**FIG. 20-1d**

### BENEFITS

Develops the muscles of the shoulders, upper arms and forearms.
Strengthens wrists and hands.
Builds endurance.

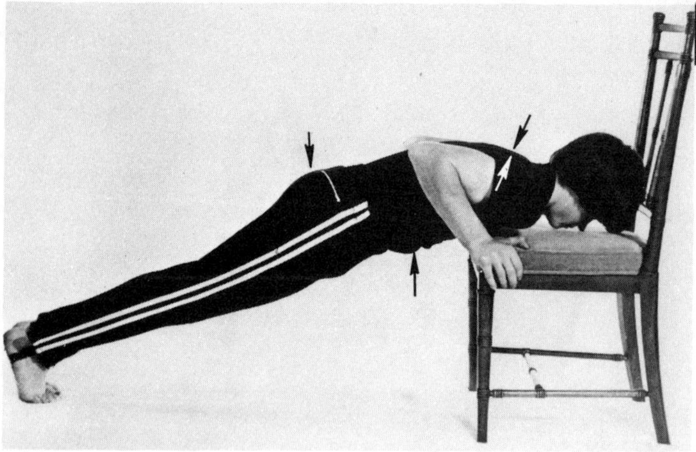

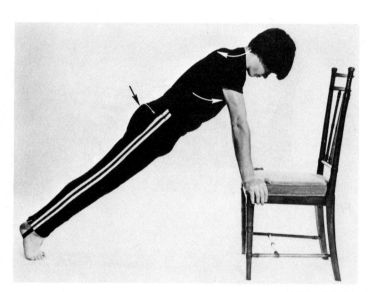

FIG. 20-2a

FIG. 20-2b

## Push-Up With Chair

### TECHNIQUE

1. Kneel in front of a chair; place your hands on the edge, and lower your shoulders so they are directly over the hands. Curl your toes under.

2. Inhale, extending sternum, raise your knees and kneecaps, tighten the buttocks, bringing yourself into a straight incline. Keep your abdomen in as you create a shoulder blade squeeze, away from the ears *(FIG. 20-2a)*.

3. Exhale, maintaining a straight line, and straighten your arm to push yourself up *(FIG. 20-2b)*. Keep that blade squeeze.

4. Inhale, extending the sternum and maintaining a straight line as you lower yourself down, leading from the sternum, not from your nose.

5. Repeat as often as you wish, but stop if you lose your alignment.

## Push-Ups

### TECHNIQUE

1. Lie face down with palms beside the chest and fingers in line with the shoulders.
2. Inhaling, curl your toes under. Without moving toes, knees or hands, exhale, pushing with your arms, raise your buttocks, chest, and head from the floor, until arms are straight.
3. With toes stationary, inhale, tighten your buttocks and bring yourself up to a straight incline *(FIG. 20-2c)*.
4. Exhaling, lower your sternum and make a blade squeeze down away from the neck. Feel the aligned spine!
5. Inhale, concentrate on the strength and control you have in your arms. With tightened buttocks, exhale, and slowly lower your straight body until chest barely touches the floor *(FIG. 20-2d)*. Lead with your sternum as you lower, not with your head; keep neck relaxed.
6. Supporting yourself only on hands and toes, inhale, push your body and legs up into a straight line by straightening your arms until they are fully extended.
7. If needed, adjust shoulder blades. Repeat the above as often as you wish, but stop if you lose your alignment.

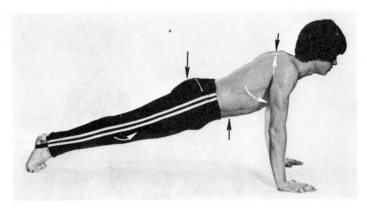

**FIG. 20-2c**

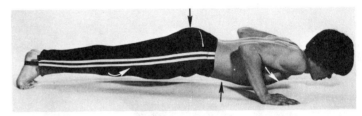

**FIG. 20-2d**

### TIPS

1. Remember to push down with the heel of your hand; tip your pelvis keeping abdomen in. It must not sag.
2. Hold body straight throughout. Keep away from common fault of lifting buttocks up high; keep them tight.
3. You must lead from the sternum as you lower your body, not from the nose.
4. Aim for consecutive push-ups, without touching the floor with your chest. Only lower as far as you can maintain control and alignment, and push up from that point.

### BENEFITS

Develops muscles of the arms, shoulders and chest.
Strengthens waist and hands.
Builds endurance.

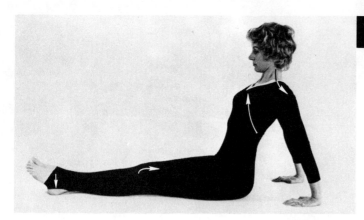

FIG. 20-3a

### TECHNIQUE

1. Sit on the floor with legs straight in front. Leaning back, place the palms on the floor behind the hips, with your fingers pointing toward your feet from approximately 6 inches in back of hips. See **FIG. 20-3a.**

2. Inhale, extend sternum, preparing to take the pressure of the body on the hands and feet. Exhaling, tighten and lift the buttocks and legs from the floor, so your soles are flat on the floor and body is in a straight incline.

3. Straighten your arms and legs, keeping the knees and elbows tightened **(FIG. 20-3b).**

4. Inhaling, extend sternum and elongate. Exhale as you shrug your shoulders down toward the floor, creating a shoulder blade squeeze. Do not hunch. Elongate the back of the neck, lightly tucking in the chin.

5. Inhale, extending sternum, and elongate further. Exhale, keeping the neck free, and tighten the buttocks as you raise hips higher.

6. Continue to breathe in rhythm with this motion for 3 breaths, gaining a balance within this pose. Only then do I want you to continue.

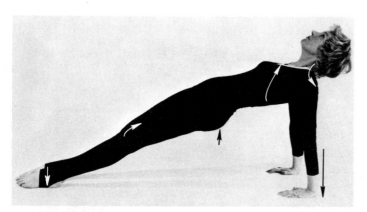

FIG. 20-3b

7. Inhaling, check neck position, extend sternum, and elongate. Exhaling, tighten buttocks and lift hips high as you press the left foot onto the floor. This enables you to raise the right leg *(FIG. 20-3c).* While up there, inhale; then exhale while you tighten buttocks and lift your hips.

8. Slowly lower the leg to the floor, and repeat with the left leg.

9. From *FIG. 20-3b* position, inhale, extend sternum and elongate. Exhale as you turn to the left, lowering the left hip to the floor *(FIG. 20-3d).*

10. Inhaling, elongate and lift yourself by reaching with the hips to *FIG. 20-3b.*

11. Then repeat Step 9 and 10 on the right side.

12. Lie down and relax. You deserve it.

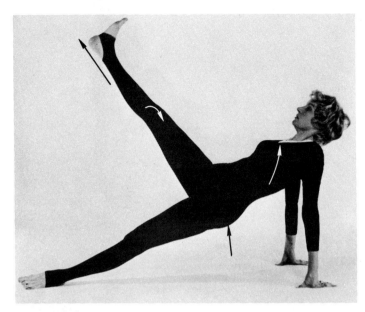

**FIG. 20-3c**

*TIPS*

1. Take care not to hunch your shoulders toward your ears. Keep shoulders shrugged down and back, creating that shoulder Blade Squeeze.

2. You may relax after each variation.

3. If you get cramps in your feet, don't point your toes, just press your heels onto the floor, keeping your toes relaxed.

4. It is very helpful to have your feet on something so they will not slide.

5. You can go up by placing the whole palm down with fingers in the direction of the feet or away from the body, as in FIGS. 20-3a and b. Another way is to lift up onto your thumbs (FIGS. 20-3c and d).

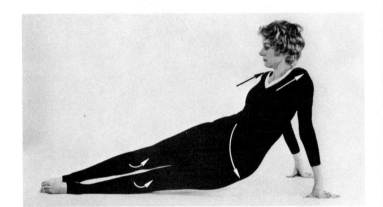

**FIG. 20-3d**

*BENEFITS*

Reduces excess weight and greatly strengthens, develops, and streamlines the legs, thighs, and buttocks.
Limbers the spine and shoulders.
Improves balance.
Strengthens arms and wrists.

## SIDE INCLINED PLANE POSE

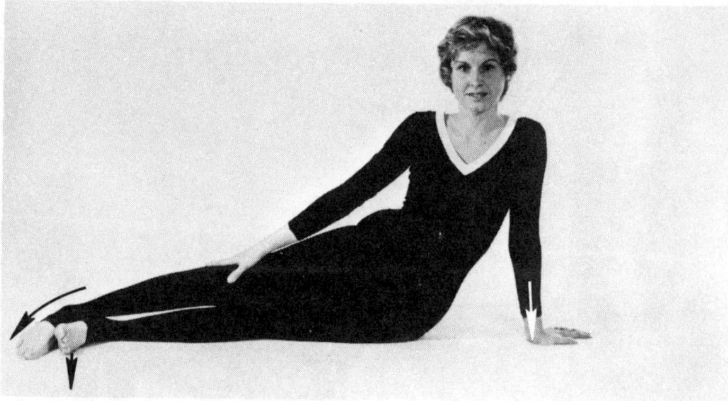

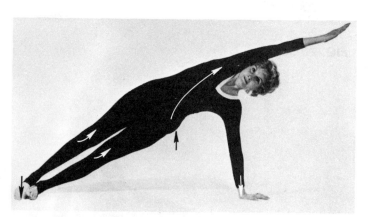

*FIG. 20-4a*

*FIG. 20-4b*

### *TECHNIQUE*

1. Sit on your left side, leaning back on your hand which is facing away from the body. Place the right hand on the thigh. Bring your body into a straight line ***(FIG. 20-4a).***
2. Make sure your wrist is directly under your shoulder. Extend your left heel, bringing your toes forward ***(FIG. 20-4a).*** The outer side of the right foot should rest firmly on the floor. Place the right ankle over the left foot. Press the ball of the right foot firmly onto the floor to keep the left foot from sliding.
3. Inhale, extend your sternum as you elongate. For leverage, push your left palm onto the floor as you raise your hip and leg from the floor. As you go up, also raise your right arm overhead ***(FIG. 20-4b).***
4. Take 3 breaths in this position to realign your balance. While doing so, check that your kneecaps are raised, buttocks are tightened, and you keep extending from the ribs reaching with the straight arm. Keep your right arm touching your ear.

5. When you feel secure in this position, you may exhale, bending the right leg at the knee and catching the right foot with the right hand *(FIG. 20-4c)*. Keep aligned.

6. Now inhale, pulling the right arm and leg up vertically *(FIG. 20-4d)*. Keep the arms and legs straight, buttocks tight, and the body in the correct alignment; do not sag.

7. To come down, keep hold of the right foot as you lower your hip to the floor. Then let go of the foot and replace it on top of the left foot. Bring yourself up to a straight sitting position with legs and back straight, grasping the balls of the feet. Lower yourself toward the floor in a Forward Bend and relax before repeating on the opposite side.

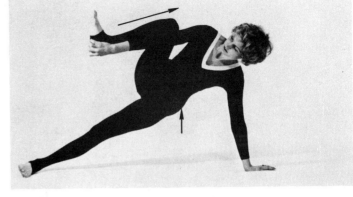

**FIG. 20-4c**

### TIPS

1. If your mat surface will cause you to slide, you may place the inner side of your left foot against a wall.

2. Before you attempt Steps 5–6, check your leg flexibility by sitting as in FIG. 20-4a. Bend the right knee so you can clasp the foot to see if you can straighten it out.

3. It is very important to distribute your weight evenly between the side of your heel and the side of the ball of your foot.

4. Be aware of the necessity for the breathing rhythm and the concentrated effect on the abdomen muscles for balance.

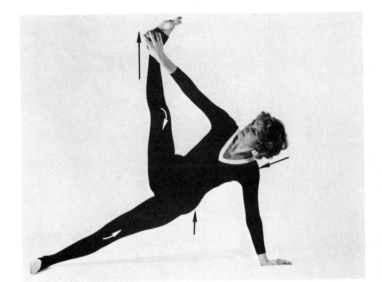

**FIG. 20-4d**

### BENEFITS

Firms thigh, calf and buttocks.
Strengthens arms and wrists.
Promotes balance.

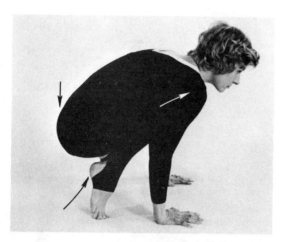

**FIG. 20-5a**

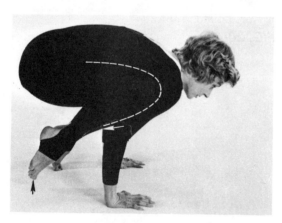

**FIG. 20-5b**

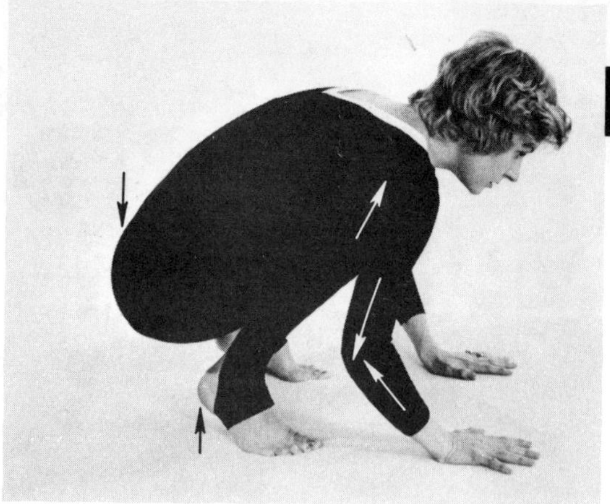

### TECHNIQUE

1. Crouch as in **FIG. 20-5a,** with feet hip-distance apart. Place hands on floor in front of feet, fingers pointing forward with the proper "Hand Grip." Make sure that your knees are up as high on the arms as possible and behind the shoulders. When you have reached this point, wing out your elbows **(FIG. 20-5a)**. Inhale as you extend your sternum.

2. Exhaling, lean forward on your toes, bringing them to a pointed position. Keep the buttocks low **(FIG. 20-5b)**.

3. Keep leaning forward until you can bring your elbows in to form a straight vertical line with your forearm **(FIG. 20-5c)**. Keeping the toes pointed will form a firm calf.

4. The calf muscles rest on the shelf formed by your upper arm. The pressure of contact is felt only on the calf muscle, not across the shin bone. Raise 1 foot at a time, keeping toes pointed **(FIG. 20-5c)**.

5. Inhale, extending sternum and looking within your range of vision. Exhale, and—believe it or not—create a slight shoulder blade squeeze. **(FIG. 20-5d)**. This will help your balance.

6. Hold for the count of 5. Slowly come out of it, and repeat if you wish.

**FIG. 20-5c**
**FIG. 20-5d**

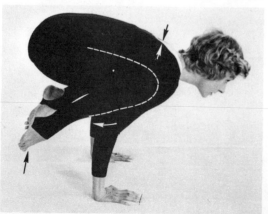

### TIPS

1. Throughout this pose the knee is always challenging the upper arm.
2. If you fear falling forward, it may reassure you to place a pillow in front of you.
3. To maintain the proper balance, keep your toes pointed after they have left the floor.
4. Do not kick up. Review Steps 3–5 carefully.

### BENEFITS

Develops poise.
Strengthens arms.
Firms legs and thighs.

### TECHNIQUE

1. Crouch down on your toes, with your chest to the left side of your left thigh. Place both hands on the floor to the left of your feet *(FIG. 20-6a)*.

2. Exhale as you lean into the right arm, placing the right elbow under the left thigh. The knee rests on the back of the upper right arm as close to the armpit as possible *(FIG. 20-6b)*. Take a few breaths here.

3. Exhale and firmly press both palms down to the floor, look within your range of vision, and raise both legs to be almost parallel to the floor, while balancing on your right upper arm, as in *FIG. 20-6c*. Hold for a count of 5 and repeat to the other side. Relax for a few moments.

4. For a variation, you can cross the left leg over the right at the ankle. Place your right hand and elbow between the legs.

5. Bend the right elbow back to support you under the right thigh. Exhale as you lean forward and onto the right upper arm. Raise the feet from the floor *(FIG. 20-6d)*. Hold for the count of 5 and slowly lower yourself to the floor. Relax.

6. Repeat to the other side.

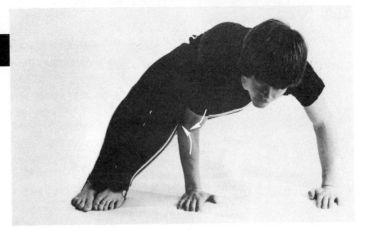

**FIG. 20-6a**

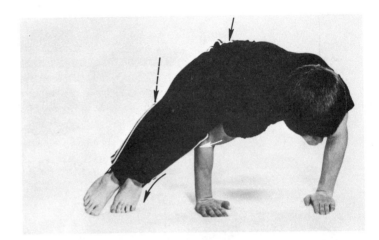

**FIG. 20-6b**

### TIPS

1. Before you try the Raven Pose, make sure you can accomplish the Crow Pose in the previous posture.

2. While you work your way into this pose, observe your "Range of Vision."

3. In order to accomplish this posture it is important to have your elbow in far enough under your thigh.

4. Surprisingly, the greatest pressure is felt in the right wrist, which is apparently free.

### BENEFITS

Improves balance and coordination.
Strengthens wrists and arms.
Tones legs.

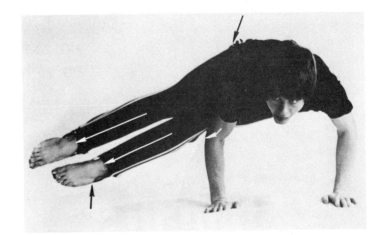

**FIG. 20-6c**
**FIG. 20-6d**

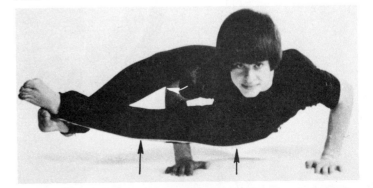

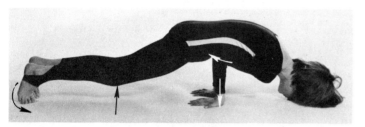

FIG. 20-7a

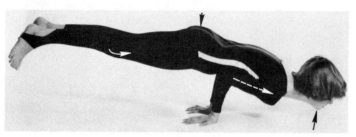

FIG. 20-7b

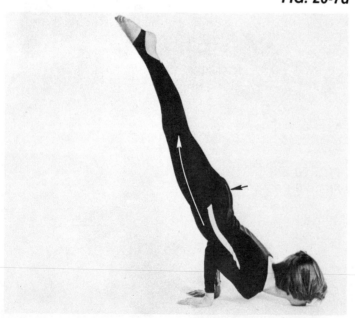

FIG. 20-7c
FIG. 20-7d

### TECHNIQUE

1. Kneel down, forehead on the floor in front of you. Arms are between the legs, hands together with the fingers, pointing toward the toes. Inhale, bend your fingers, pointing toward the toes. Inhale, bend your elbows and walk forward on your knees. Exhale while you try to get your elbows together, working them down as far as possible below the navel *(FIG. 20-7a)*. You may attempt to get them lower, but the average place is inside and level with the hip bones.

2. Rest the forehead on the floor and straighten your legs until you are supported by your head, hands, and toes, bearing the body weight on the wrists and hands *(FIG. 20-7b)*.

3. Inhale as you lean forward slightly, raising your feet and head simultaneously until the body arches up from the floor. You are balancing on your upper arms *(FIG. 20-7c)*. Exhale and come down slowly. Rest, and take a couple of deep breaths.

4. Now try this! Keep your chin on the floor, still leaning forward, tighten your buttocks, and exhale as you raise your legs all the way up *(FIG. 20-7d)*.

5. Slowly lower yourself to the floor, remove the arm and relax.

### TIPS

1. Do take the time to work your elbows as far below the navel as possible, almost to the pelvic bones.

2. Once you have placed your elbows in the proper position, do not let them slip away. It is the placement of the elbows that will give the proper balance for raising all of the legs.

### BENEFITS

Strengthens the back and abdominal muscles. Improves digestion and tones up all vital organs. Stimulates the flow of blood to the head.

# 21 BREATHING TECHNIQUES

"And the Lord God formed man of the dust of the ground, and breathed into his nostrils the breath of life, and man became a living soul." (Genesis 2:7). All life is breath and without breath there is no life.

Pranayama is the Yogic system of breath control. In translation it means simply the control of the vital energy, Life-Force, the air we breathe. The seat and storage place of vital energy in the body is the solar plexus (the upper middle part of the abdomen). There are many breathing exercises which direct "prana" to this center, and others which send it to different parts of the body—the glands, vital organs, nervous plexuses—with recharging and re-vitalizing effects. In most cases the breathing exercises themselves are very easy to perform. The really difficult part is to control the mind and train it to work with and for you.

I recommend that you practice the following postures with the supervision of an *experienced* teacher.

1. Always practice in a well ventilated room without drafts.

2. Wear loose, comfortable clothing.

3. Practice on a stomach that is empty of all except light liquids. Never practice vigorous breathing until an hour or two has elapsed after a light meal, and two to three hours after a heavier meal.

4. Light food can be taken half an hour after finishing.

5. Before starting, the bowels and bladder should be emptied.

6. You must sit with back absolutely erect, with the complete spine perpendicular to the floor.

7. There should be no strain felt in the facial muscles, eyes, ears, neck, shoulders, or arms. If in the Lotus, deliberately relax the legs and feet.

8. Eyes should be closed when possible, for, if kept open, a burning sensation and irritability might be felt.

9. Throughout practice, the brain is kept passive but alert. The ear listens for the proper sound of the breath. The hand and throat are used to observe or control the breath flow.

10. The student must be alert and sensitive to the flow of prana within him, while he is conscious of time, posture, and maintaining an even breath rhythm.

11. Each student should measure his own capacity and not exceed it. Capacity is reached when the smooth rhythm of breathing is lost.

12. A healthy body and sound mind can be shaken by faulty practice.

13. Never practice the asanas right after pranayama. Let an hour elapse. However, pranayama can be done shortly after a mild practice session.

14. Persons suffering from high blood pressure or heart trouble should never attempt to hold their breath in after an inhalation. They can practice Alternate Breathing without the retention and gain beneficial effects.

15. Persons suffering from low blood pressure can do Alternate Breathing with retention after inhalation *only*, with beneficial effects. They should not retain breath after exhalation.

16. Conditions that preclude Bhastrika or Kapalabhati:
    A) Poor lung capacity
    B) Ear or eye complaints
    C) High or low blood pressure

17. Care should be taken not to bloat the abdomen in the process of inhalation, during all the types of Pranayama.

18. Except for Alternate Breathing, which *can* be done every day, the following breathing exercises are not to be done all in one session. You should alternate the days for each.

19. Do not overdo it. Pranayama is not complicated, but it is very concentrated, so be careful. After any forced breathing, always have a period in your relaxed natural rhythm to stabilize yourself.

Alternate Breathing consists of deep controlled breathing through each nostril to bring purification of the nerves. It usually is practiced following the postures, or just before relaxation, and is a vital part of our Yoga routine. When we do this exercise, we are to concentrate on exhaling completely—letting out all the carbon dioxide. When we inhale, we replenish our body with a flow of fresh oxygen which we hold for awhile to allow for absorption into the system.

The finger placement can be your choice. In **DIAGRAM 1** the index and middle fingers are turned down so the thumb and ring finger are close to the nose with little finger next to the ring finger.

In **DIAGRAM 2,** both fingers are placed on the space between the eyebrows, leaving the other fingers free to close the nose; with this placement, you can focus the attention on one area.

Shall we begin?

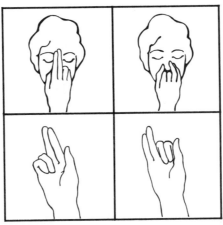

**Diagram 1**        **Diagram 2**

## TECHNIQUE

1. Sit with an erect spine, eyes closed.
2. Completely exhale from both nostrils.
3. Close the right nostril with the right thumb.
4. Draw in the air very slowly through the left nostril.
5. Close the left nostril with the ring and little fingers of the right hand. (Both nostrils now closed.)
6. Pause. Remove your thumb, and exhale slowly through the right nostril.
7. Inhale slowly through the same side (right nostril).
8. Close both nostrils and pause.
9. Remove your ring and little fingers, and exhale slowly through the left nostril.
10. This constitutes 1 round. Start with 5 rounds and gradually increase the number to 10 rounds.

### Variations

1. Begin with equal units of breathing in and out rhythmically. Starting from 5 counts, working to 10 counts. This is called the "purifying breath."
2. If you have practiced the "purifying breath" for awhile and feel comfortable in it, you may increase your exhalation ratio, working up to 5–10. Advance only if you can maintain a smooth rhythm.

3. After you achieve mastery over the 5–10 ratio, you may apply a retention between breaths. Start from a ratio of 5–10 and work gradually to 5–20–10. It is not necessary to carry this further. The ratio should be increased only as long as it is comfortable.

4. This precision is achieved only after long practice. Do not attempt it all at once.

5. Experienced students only may apply the Mula Bandha during retention after inhalation. This contracts the anal sphincter muscle, pulling up the lower abdomen toward the diaphragm.

6. Do not attempt to hold your breath after exhalation until you have mastered the 5–20–10 ratio. Make sure you are under the guidance of an experienced teacher.

7. When done correctly and with caution, Alternate Breathing excercises are beneficial in soothing frayed nerves, and bring about a sense of tranquility.

## KAPALABHATI PRANAYAMA

Kapalabhati means "that which makes the skull shine" and definitely has an activating effect. The body is vitalized, and the solar plexus is strengthened and recharged with vital energy.

### TECHNIQUE

1. Take a deep inhalation and then a vigorous exhalation. After each rapid exhalation, relax the abdominal muscles and immediately fill the lower and middle part of the lungs with air.
2. The air is snorted out through the nose by creating short, sharp contractions with the abdomen.
3. The rapid bellows-like exhalation must be made in quick succession through a vigorous tensing of the abdominal muscles.
4. Immediately repeat, inhale, and again vigorously exhale.
5. The inhalation should be twice as long as the exhalation.
6. Continue repeating this ratio until the snorting lessens and makes you comfortably tired. Lie down and relax.

## BHASTRIKA PRANAYAMA

Bhastrika means "bellows" (as used in a furnace). The air is forcibly drawn in and forced out as in a blacksmith's bellows.

### Stage I

### TECHNIQUE

1. Begin by taking a fast, vigorous breath, and then exhale sharply and forcefully. This completes 1 cycle.
2. Make the sound resemble air rushing through bellows. Repeat for 10 cycles.
3. Then take a slow deep breath, completely filling the lungs, but do not distend the abdomen. Hold a second or two, tightening the anal muscle. Then slowly and deeply exhale.
4. Step 3 rests the lungs and the diaphragm and prepares them for a fresh cycle.

5. Repeat the 10 cycles of Bhastrika 3–4 times with the Complete Breath in between.

6. If the sound lessens and the vigor diminishes, then reduce their number.

7. When completed, lie down and relax.

## Stage II

### TECHNIQUE

1. Apply the above technique, but use the alternate nostril breath instead of both nostrils.

2. Close the left nostril, keeping the right nostril open.

3. Employ the 10 cycles of Bhastrika through the right nostril, as in Stage I.

4. Close the right nostril and open the left, repeating the 10 cycles with the left nostril.

5. Release the fingers. Take a few deep Complete Breaths.

6. Repeat the cycles on both sides 3–4 times with the Complete Breath in between.

7. When completed, lie down and relax.

### BENEFITS

Kapalabhati is not as strenuous as Bhastrika.

Kapalabhati and Bhastrika activate and invigorate the liver, pancreas, spleen and abdominal muscles.

Aids in digestion and warms the body.

Counteracts the effects of asthma and drains sinuses.

The Uddiyana Bandha means the "restraint of the flying-up impulses," better known as the Abdominal Lift. It is marvelous for energyzing the body. Drawing in the abdominal muscles causes the thorax to expand, while forcing the viscerae and diaphragm upward until a large hollow cavity appears under the ribs.

The prana or energy is made to move from the lower abdomen toward the head.

To practice, make sure you have an empty stomach and emptied both the bladder and the bowels. It helps to practice in front of a mirror in your underwear.

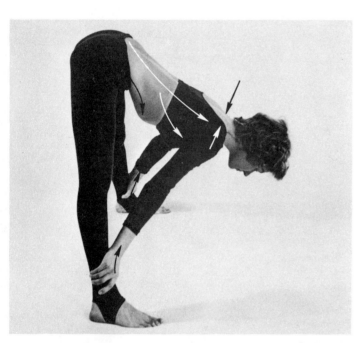

FIG. 21-1a

## TECHNIQUE

1. Stand with legs completely apart.
2. Take 3 deep complete Rib-Cage Breaths.
3. On the exhalation of the third, bend forward, blowing out the air with a strong and forcible expiration (then "Ha" the rest out as you bend down to grasp your ankles, as in **FIG. 21-1a).**
4. Wait until your lungs are completely emptied. At this point, close the mouth, press the tongue against the roof of the mouth, and use this "valve" to lock the breath out.
5. It is most important that no breath be in the body throughout this exercise. Without inhaling, but performing a *mock* inhalation, extend the sternum and pull the tummy in and up, as in **FIG. 21-1a.**
6. Raise your head up, bend the knees, place your hands high up on the thighs without hunching your shoulders, and tip your pelvis, as in **FIG. 21-1d.**
7. Without breathing, pull the abdomen further inward and upward with a suction action, which will expand the thorax, thus raising the diaphragm, as high as possible, as in **FIG. 21-b.** If properly performed, you will feel a strong pull at the base of the throat because of the vacuum created in your lungs.

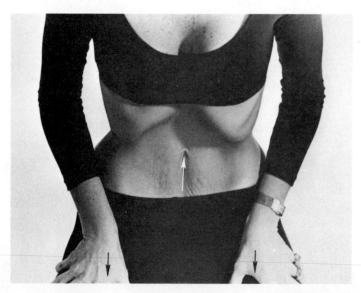

FIG. 21-1b

8. When you have learned to suck in your abdomen (as if to press the navel against the backbone, as in **FIG. 21-1c,** endeavor to lift abdomen up toward the breastbone, pressing the hands against the thighs, as in **FIG. 21-1d.**

9. Hold the inward pull for one second before letting the abdomen drop down by itself. *Do not push it out.* Immediately pull the abdomen in and up again, still keeping the breath out, and then let it drop.

10. Repeat this in, up, and out motion for a total of 3–5 times on the single exhalation.

11. Relax with a slow inhalation and take 2 more Rib-Cage Breaths to equalize your breathing again.

12. Perform the above set of 3–5 contractions 3 times, taking time to normalize the breathing in between. In the beginning, I suggest only 1 set of 3 contractions.

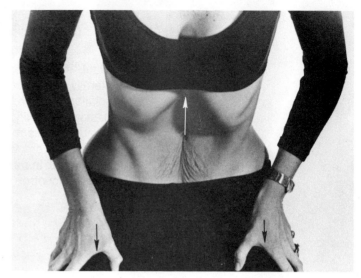

**FIG. 21-1c**

## TIPS

1. It helps to create a greater vacuum if you tighten the anal sphincter muscle when creating the suction.

2. Do not look at your abdomen. You will cut off the suction in the throat. Do look straight ahead into the mirror. You will be able to see the vacuum at both the abdomen and the base of the throat and then feel it.

3. The muscles of the abdominal wall must be relaxed and must remain passive; if contracted, they work against the action of the atmospheric pressure.

4. The mock thoracic inspiration is responsible for drawing the diaphragm up to its highest level.

5. To find your personal position or stance, tilt the upper body forward only until the diaphragm pops upward. You are then in proper position to proceed. You can see the raising of the diaphragm by noticing an increase in the hollow under the ribs.

## BENEFITS

Good for circulation.

Strengthens and firms abdominal muscles, also reducing the waistline.

Excellent remedy for prolapses of the stomach, intestines, uterus, etc.

Promotes regularity and relieves constipation.

I cannot say enough for the benefits of the Abdominal Lift.

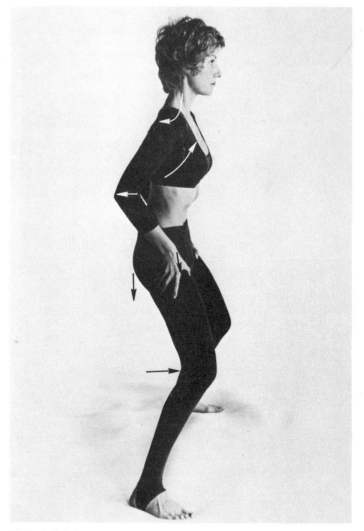

**FIG. 21-1d**

"Nauli" means that the abdominal muscles and organs are made to move laterally and vertically in a surging motion. It could also be called a central isolation of the rectus abdominal muscle. Before attempting the Nauli, first master the Uddiyana Bandha. Nauli is one of the most difficult exercises, because in this movement the rectus abdominis and the other muscles are pushed forward while contracted so that they form a ridge in front of the abdomen. In this exercise, too, these muscles must be made responsive to our voluntary control. This is not recommended for the average student.

### TECHNIQUE

1. Apply the technique of the Uddiyana Bandha through to Step 8.
2. The rectus abdominis muscles are rooted in the pit of the abdomen, just above the pubic bone.
3. Separate and contract them, forming a hard column right up the center of the abdomen.
4. Contract them to the right leaning to the right, then contract to the left leaning to the left, making the column on the appropriate side of the body. The pressure of your hand on left knee as you lean will assist in isolating these muscles.
5. Perform this action quickly (center, left, center, right, center, left, center, etc., one after another). Remember it helps to alternate corresponding hand pressure.
6. Work in a continuous churning movement, which is a series of closely integrated contractions.
7. Everything is confined to the abdominal muscles; the hips are not rotated.
8. Maintain this action and position from 5–10 seconds, according to your capacity.
9. Relax the grip, release the abdomen and inhale slowly.
10. Take a few deep breaths. Repeat the cycle 6 times. Remember, if uncomfortable, stop.
11. Practice this only once every 24 hours.

### TIPS

1. The Nauli can be learned in several weeks, while in other cases several months may be necessary for mastery.
2. You may alter your stance to gain better leverage.
3. Do not look at your abdomen. Look straight ahead into a mirror.

### BENEFITS

The deep-seated back muscles are strengthened and rejuvenated by the abundant flow of blood.

Massages all the organs of the abdominal cavity.

The organs are stimulated and brought into equilibrium.

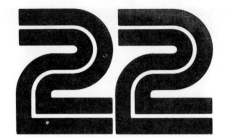

# LOTUS-RELATED POSTURES

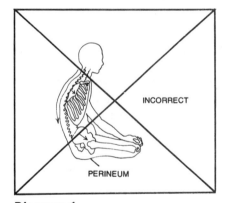

**Diagram 1**

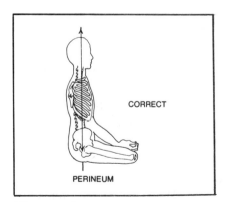

**Diagram 2**

Many Westerners on hearing the word "Yoga" visualize someone sitting in what appears to them to be an impossible posture, the Lotus. This posture, which so symbolizes the discipline of Hatha Yoga, is referred to as the prince of asanas, for it is the key position to be assumed during the Pranayama (breathing exercises).

There are two distinct health advantages to be gained from the Lotus: 1) a shift of circulation, which occurs by compelling hip and knee joints to forced flexion, allowing blood from the limbs to flow into the abdomen in greater supply, thereby increasing access of blood to the visceral organs, and 2) sitting with the body solidly based on a triangle (formed by the thighs and perineum, with the spine perfectly perpendicular) gives the student a perfect sense of psychosomatic equilibrium.

The Lotus is a difficult posture for most Westerners, and most particularly for those who start Hatha Yoga in adult life, when the lower limbs are stiffened from years of sedentary living. The pelvic girdle is often disabled because of injury, misalignment, or inadequate motion. It is helpful, therefore, to do preliminary moves which will lead to the ultimate execution of the Lotus.

Before any exercise where the knees are to be severely bent, as in the Lotus, take time to relax them by rubbing the sides of both knees vigorously with the palms. This allows the bursae to lubricate, protecting the knees from sudden forcible flexion. The aim of Lotus warm-ups is to increase movement in hip and knee joints and stretch the thighs. Therefore, exercises where you work both inward and outward rotation are helpful in augmenting the multi-directional range of motion in the hips.

When you come out of the Lotus, straighten the leg, raise the kneecap, and pull the toes toward the body, so as to elongate the hamstring and relieve any cramps that you might have encountered.

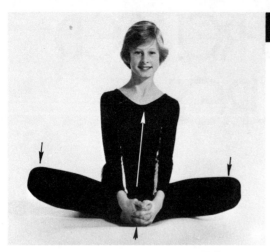

FIG. 22-1a

### Butterfly

*TECHNIQUE*

1. Sitting tall, bring soles of feet together and cup the feet with interlaced fingers. Pull against feet for leverage.
2. Inhale, elongate, extending sternum. Exhale, creating a blade squeeze. Concave the spine and work to lower the thighs *(FIG. 22-1a)*. Then continue lowering them to the floor.
3. Take several deep breaths in rhythm with this motion, then come out of it and proceed.
4. If it is too difficult to keep your back straight, sit closely up against a wall. With feet together and hands on knees, inhale elongating the spine up the wall, exhale as you shrug shoulders back and apply slight pressure to the knees lowering legs down. Don't force. Repeat breathing pattern and slight pressure about six times.

### Toe To Face

*TECHNIQUE*

1. Sit tall, bending your left leg so you can interlace your fingers around the left foot.
2. Inhale, elongate, extending sternum. Exhale as you pull the foot toward you, trying to keep the thigh close to your body and working the knee beyond your back.
3. Inhale to reinforce the elongation. Exhale as you bring the toe to touch the forehead, nose and chin, as in *FIG. 22-1b*.

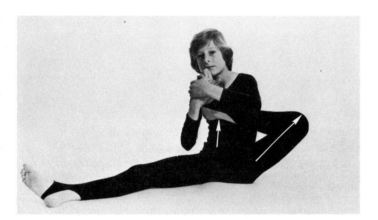

FIG. 22-1b

### The Cradle

*TECHNIQUE*

1. Keeping the left foot up high, place it into the crook of the right arm. Bring the left arm around and interlace the hands, creating your cradle. *(FIG. 22-1c)*.
2. Inhale, elongate, extending sternum to straighten your back. Exhale as you rock the leg from right to left.
3. Inhale, elongating again. Exhale, this time hugging the leg close to your chest. Hold, feeling the stretch in the thigh.

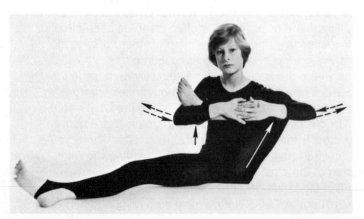

FIG. 22-1c

## Talk The Knee Down

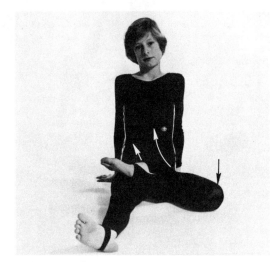

**FIG. 22-1d**

### TECHNIQUE

1. Keeping the foot high and close to the body, take hold of foot with your hands.

2. Turn the foot around so the sole is facing you. Place the instep up high on the thigh as you lower the knee to the floor. The closer you bring the heel to the hip bone, the less pressure on the instep.

3. Lean back on your hands. Inhale, extending sternum. Exhale as you "talk" the knee down **(FIG. 22-1d).** Do not push it down. If the knee drops easily, keep it there and—would you believe—tip your pelvis.

4. Take several deep breaths, working the knee down. Hold for a few moments with it down, but do not use your hands.

5. Slowly straighten out the leg and pull on the foot working toes toward you to stretch out the hamstrings. Then, repeat with other leg.

### TIPS

1. It is very beneficial if you spend the time on a warm-up of the knees before you begin. Bend the left knee toward the chest and rub the side of the knee with open palms. Rub virgorously using a rotating motion. Now press the back of the knee with your fingers as you bend the knee to your chest. Hold a few moments; release. Lower the leg to the floor. Work with the fingertips to lift and move the knee cap. All of this will warm up the knee.

2. Do not force your thigh, knee, or foot in any of these positions. Advance gradually.

3. Unless you can "talk" the knee to the floor (as in FIG. 22-1d), you must not attempt a Lotus. Just keep working with the warm-ups. In time, you will be able to accomplish the Lotus with comfort.

### BENEFITS

Develops flexibility in the hips.
Tones thighs, knees and feet.
Prepares you for the Lotus.

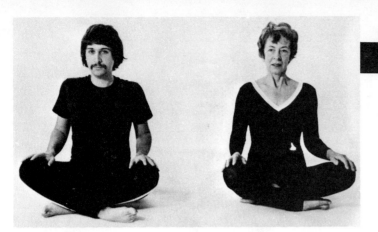

FIG. 22-2a

### Easy Posture

*TECHNIQUE*

1. Sit tall. Bend your right leg, and place the right foot under your left knee. Bend your left leg, placing the left foot under the right knee, as in *FIG. 22-2a* (left). You are in an easy comfortable cross-legged position. Head and back should be kept in a straight line without sagging.

2. If you find this uncomfortable and difficult, sit up against a wall. Fold a large (beach) towel thick enough to place under you so you will be able to bring your feet under with a mimimum of discomfort. To ease the pressure place small folded towels above your feet. Inhale as you elongate the spine and as you exhale don't slouch—keep the sternum erect, relaxing the shoulders.

### Crossed Ankles

*TECHNIQUE*

Sit tall. Bend your right leg, and place the right heel on the floor up high against the thigh. Bend the left leg, placing the left foot under the right leg as in *FIG. 22-a* (right).

### Ankles Side By Side

FIG. 22-2b

*TECHNIQUE*

Sit, bend your left leg, bringing your left heel up close to the crotch. Bend your right leg, and place the right foot in front of the left foot, with toes along the shin bone, as in *FIG. 22-2b* (left).

### Half-Lotus

*TECHNIQUE*

1. Sit, bending the left leg at the knee, holding the left foot with your hands. Turn the foot around so the sole is facing you. Place the instep up high on the thigh as you lower the knee to the floor. The higher you bring the heel toward the hip bone, the less pressure on the instep.

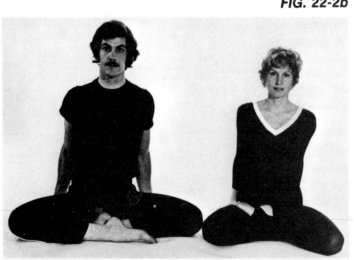

2. Bend your right leg and place it under the left thigh, as in **FIG. 22-b** (right).

## Slipped Lotus

### TECHNIQUE

1. Repeat the techniques of Step 1, Half-Lotus.
2. Let the first foot slip as you bend your other leg. Hold the foot with your hands and place it over the thigh. Let the feet slip down until the ankle touches the floor and the heels meet, as in **FIG. 22-2c** (left).

## Beginner's Lotus

### TECHNIQUE

1. Sit, bend your left leg, holding the left foot with your hands. Turn the foot around so the sole is facing you. Place the instep up high on the thigh as you lower the knee to the floor.
2. Bend the right leg. Holding the right foot with your hands, place the instep up high on the left thigh, as in **FIG. 22-2c** (right).

## Intermediate Lotus

### TECHNIQUE

1. Repeat the techniques of the Beginner's Lotus, Steps 1-2, but work to bring the heels up higher and closer to the hip bones while you bring the thighs closer together, as in **FIG. 22-2d** (left).

## Advanced Lotus

### TECHNIQUE

1. Repeat the techniques of the Intermediate Lotus, but this time, really work to bring your heels up high, and work to bring thighs parallel.
2. To accomplish the Bound Lotus, exhale, swing the right arm back from the shoulders and bring the hand near the left hip. Catch the right big toe, hold the position, and inhale.
3. Exhaling, repeat the above, using the left arm to grab the left toes, as in **FIG. 22-2d** (right).
4. To aid in the grip, shrug the shoulders back so that the shoulder blades are brought close to each other and the chest is expanded forward.

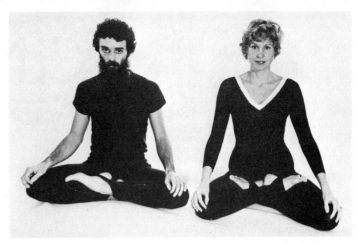

**FIG. 22-2c**

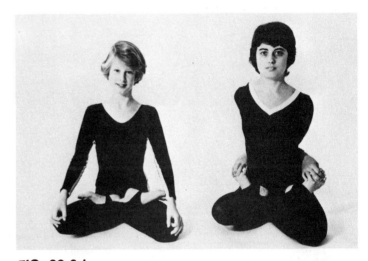

**FIG. 22-2d**

### TIPS

1. Do not force yourself in these positions, but *do* spend time warming up properly.
2. Do not slouch. It is important to sit up directly on the ischium bones. Inhale as you extend the sternum, elongating the spine. Exhale, as you balance the shoulders and concave the spine. Maintain a continuous lift of the spine from the hip girdle.
3. Do not always favor the same side as you go into these positions. Reverse the process by starting with the opposite leg. It is good to equalize muscle tone and flexibility.
4. After you have accomplished any of the variations above, relax the leg with a Forward Bend stretch.

### BENEFITS

Relieves stiffness in knees and ankles.
The spine and abdominal organs are toned.
Aligns the spine and keeps the mind attentive and alert.

# 23 RELAXATION

INCORRECT

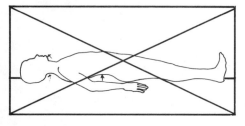

CORRECT

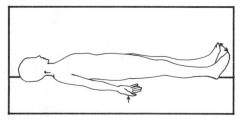

Relaxation is a kind of physical and mental "letting go." This must come naturally and cannot be forced. Ideally, one should be able to maintain the "letting go" feeling at all times, for it is in this state that one's best work is done. But unfortunately most people consider relaxation as something which is supposed to be done at a specific time. Americans are finding it more and more difficult to let go even when they are supposed to be relaxing and having a good time.

We recognize the problem of tension within ourselves and around us. The pace of life, current world conditions, constant movement through travel, highly developed forms of enjoyment, and television and the stereo boom all tend to make us function with brain and body at a speed that is too intense.

The term "tension" is really quite vague and there are as many feelings and definitions about this as there are people who have experienced any type of disturbance or uneasiness. Of course, tension manifests itself in these familiar symptoms: inability to slow down, relax or sleep, unstable attention span, tense nerves, and finally a growing anxiety about everything and everyone. If these tensions are not dealt with, they will in time translate themselves into physical problems: heart trouble, headaches, colitis, ulcers, indigestion, malfunctioning gall bladder, high blood pressure, hypertension, poor circulation and, very possibly, even cancer.

We might like to consider this the price paid for progress in technology, but that does not solve the problem. Yes, tension is with us today, but it has always been present under different names and is a highly individual and personal problem. In all of the political crises throughout human history, there are always those who are able to maintain their composure, dignity and serenity and be of real aid to their fellow men. You can catch "tension" from your neighbor in the same way as you can catch a cold when your physical resistance is inadequate. Conversely, you can avoid catching tensions if your level of serenity is sufficiently high.

If, because of the strength of your religious faith, you are not beset with tensions, you are probably able to maintain your tranquility. However, there are vast numbers of Americans who are suffering from anxiety and fear, which are now classified under the general term of "tension."

How can we integrate a more relaxed pace into our present way of living? First we have to learn to slow down from within. Our life-force (energy) is as close to us as our heartbeat, pulse, and respiration. By learning to control our respiration, we can monitor our feelings, emotions, and desires. The breathing process follows the pace of our activity. Strenuous emotional activity will speed up the heart, causing shallow breathing and weakening the oxygenation process until the whole system begins to feel the strain. This all happens because of a lack of harmony between our lifestyle and the basic rhythms of our breath, body and mind.

To gain this basic harmony, we have the slow movement of our Hatha Yoga postures, rhythmic breathing and the necessary discipline needed to coordinate the positions and movements within a posture.

Relaxation means slowing down our system, first physically and then mentally. For your first lesson in relaxation, consider tomorrow morning. You will rush out of bed, get dressed, and gulp down your breakfast. STOP! Sit down quietly, eat slowly, making sure to really savor and chew your food. Take time to take some rhythmic breaths between bites. Feel the tension subside and energy gained. Pick up this rhythm of awareness of motion and breathing as you go to work, driving with this same sense of calmness, not allowing the traffic to get the best of you. Remember *you* control your body; do not let life control you. Now for mid-morning and time for the awaited "coffee-break." Instead of gulping down your coffee and smoking, take an "oxygen break." Forget (even if you have only five minutes) all your immediate cares. Let them wait. What is the very worst thing that can happen if you stop and have an "oxygen break"? Why nothing. And how much better you will feel for it. Instead of smoking, take a deep drag on your breath—your life-force, energy. Take time to really relax on the exhalation. Repeat until you get in tune with yourself and are reunited with that harmony of breath and motion.

Relaxation is not a matter of will-power, but rather of enjoyment, of settling into physical patterns and using this experience to focus your strongest forces toward whatever you are doing.

Since this is a book on Hatha Yoga, you will want to know the Yoga way to relax. I am going to offer you a routine in relaxation which has been used so successfully through many centuries to achieve a high, natural level of tranquility. Through this practice, you do not force yourself to relax; you do not have to fight to "let go." This happens effortlessly, naturally, and beautifully. So let us begin.

## TECHNIQUE

1. Lie down slowly on your mat. To align your body as in **FIG. 23-1a,** tip your pelvis, extend the heels, keep feet together, and inhaling, extend the sternum and rotate the shoulders downward as you extend the arms lengthwise. Then exhale, letting the arms relax, and raise your head up and check that chin, sternum, navel, and ankles are in a straight line. Elongating the back of the neck, slowly lower the neck and head to the floor as you relax the feet. Only now are you ready for the relaxation, as shown in **FIG. 23-1b.**

2. Close your eyes and put all thoughts and distractions out of your mind. Just concentrate on yourself and be aware of how you feel. Pretend you are taking a mental sunbath.

3. Let your body gradually become limp and heavy; pretend you are slowly sinking into the floor.

4. For the first round, the rhythm will be to breathe in deeply, tense up, and then let go suddenly with a concentrated sigh.

5. Go down to the right foot; breathe in deeply as you tense it. Hold your breath, keep the foot tensed for a few seconds, and then breathe out with a sigh and release all the muscular contractions in the foot, feeling it become heavy and sink onto the floor.

6. Wait a few seconds and repeat the process with the left foot. Keep the rest of the body loose as you tense each separate part.

7. Then breathe in deeply as you tense the right leg. (Keep the left leg loose.) Hold the tension and breathe. Then release and exhale. Now repeat by tensing the left leg; hold, and let it go.

8. Tense buttocks as you inhale, and hold for a moment. (Keep the rest of the body loose.) Then release and exhale; feel yourself sinking further onto the floor.

9. Now tense the chest and shoulders as you take a nice deep inhalation. Hold, breathe, and tense (keep arm loose). Release the contraction in the chest and shoulders as you exhale. Pause.

10. Go down to the right hand, as if to hold a great big beach ball; inhaling, outstretch the fingers and hold on to the ball, gripping tighter and tighter. The back of the hand stays on the floor. Now, exhaling, let the ball go. Imagine that it has bounced into the left hand; inhale, and outstretch those fingers. Hold,

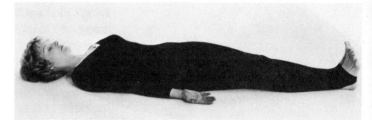

**FIG. 23-1a**

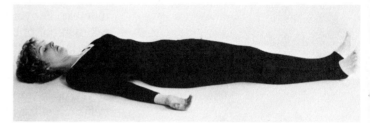

**FIG. 23-1b**

gripping tighter and tighter; now just exhale, letting it go.

11. Inhaling, elongate the neck. Exhale as you roll the head slowly to the right, taking time to lower it as far as it will go. Inhale slowly; roll up to the center. Exhale as you slowly roll to the left, hold, wait to count of 2 now. Inhale slowly, roll up to the center.

12. Take a deep breath and tense all the facial muscles, hold, exhaling, release (easing the scalp, the temple region, the forehead, the eyelids and all the facial muscles).

13. Feel your body letting go, sinking further into the mat. Concentrate now on not moving your body so that you can relax even further from within. We are going to center our attention on each particular part of the body, relaxing it without moving it.

14. Go down, concentrating on the tips of your toes; relax them by withdrawing all activity from them. In the same way, relax the arches of the feet, the heels, the ankles, the calves of the legs, the knees and thighs. Your feet and legs are now completely relaxed. Note that they feel much lighter and as if floating on your mat.

15. Now relax buttocks, hips, abdomen, and waist; relax all of them completely.

16. Going down to the lower lumbar region, relax one vertebra at a time, going up the spine.

17. When you reach the thoracic region, relax the rib cage. Your breath is now slowed down, until hardly noticeable. Let the feeling of relaxation gradually overtake the whole body.

18. Going up the spine now, relax the shoulder blades and then come around front and relax the chest. Just let those shoulders go, sinking onto the mat.

19. Going down now to the hands, feel the warmth and energy in the palms of the hands; relax them and also the wrists, elbows, upper arms, and again those shoulders and neck. Since you are not holding the head up now, relax the neck completely. Note how much lighter the head feels.

20. Focus your attention now on relaxing the scalp, temple region, and forehead; ease them completely, removing any frown lines.

21. Relax the eyelids, checkbones, nose, and lips, let them part. Drop the tongue and jaw and relax the throat.

22. Just let yourself go sinking into the mat. Be aware of how quiet and still you can be.

23. Finally relax the mind by visualizing a peace-inducing scene, for example, a beautiful garden, a deep blue sky, or soft white clouds drifting in the sky. Hold this image for some time, then dismiss it. Now imagine that you are this cloud. You feel so light, so relaxed, just floating in the sky, passing another cloud, gently gliding along, above green valleys, forests, above a small lake, and see a reflection of yourself. How refreshing to be so gentle and airy, so free and content.

24. Now dismiss all thoughts from your mind; make it completely blank, as if you were sinking into oblivion, all peaceful and quiet.

25. Remain in this state as long as you wish. Then ever so slowly, roll over on your left side with knees bent to hip level. Take 3 breaths in this position then return to your back. Awaken it by taking some deep breaths and stretching the fingers, arms, legs, and stretch the whole spine, letting yourself yawn and still stretching slowly, roll up into sitting position.

26. You have now experienced the completely relaxed state, and can do so again by yourself whenever you wish.

27. Remember, YOU control your body; do not let IT control you.

## TIPS

1. Make sure you lie on a firm flat surface with no pillow. Only if there is tension in the neck because of no pillow may you use a thin one. You might enjoy covering yourself with a big towel or blanket.

2. Take shoes off and wear loose comfortable clothing.

3. If you are going through the relaxation process and find some muscle tensing back up on you, be stern and repeatedly go back down and relax it. Remember YOU control your body.

4. Do each holding position for at least 5 seconds.

5. Concentrate fully on each part of the body you are working on. If other thoughts come in, dispassionately watch them wander past, without trying to become involved.

6. Students who wear contact lenses should refrain from tensing the eyes.

7. Perform the Sponge relaxation whenever you are tired, angry, upset, and brain-fagged. It is not a waste of time. It works!

8. If you find you need a relief and can not get into Sponge Pose, just close your eyes and take a few deep rounds of the Complete Breath, tune into the "letting go" feeling.

9. Better than the above technique is 5 rounds of Alternate Breathing. Five good concentrated rounds is as good as an hour nap.

10. Relaxation should be practiced after each exercise session in order to fully assimilate the benefits.

11. The reason this is called Sponge is that one tries to feel porous and open everywhere (like a sponge). Inhale (not just with the lungs). Visualize the life-giving energy of the surrounding atmosphere as it is being drawn in through all the limbs, providing the whole system with revitalizing power and rejuvenating every tissue of the organism.

12. Relax periodically throughout the day and you will double your efficiency. If you doubt me, then try it and see.

13. Rhythmic breathing and relaxation exercises enable you to overcome muscular tension and mental strain. Yoga can restore the normal working order of our entire organism, and the relaxation of body and mind go hand in hand with health, youth, happiness, and a long life.

# 24 YOGA TIME SCHEDULES

Beginning students can choose from amongst the following Hatha Yoga schedules, which are timed so that there is no need to rush through them. But if you find yourself rushed, please only do what you can in the correct manner, taking time for relaxation and save the remaining portion for the next day. As the student becomes more relaxed and flexible, more postures can be accomplished within the original time limit, but postures should *never* be hurried. It is a good idea to choose any extra postures from those which the student feels need more practice. Always use rhythmic breathing, and have a relaxation period at the end.

## FIVE-MINUTE PROGRAM

**1. Sun Salutation** *(p. 71)*

**2. Relaxation applying Complete Breathing**  *(pp. 208, 14)*

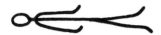

## FIFTEEN-MINUTE PROGRAM

**1. Sun Salutation**  *(p. 71)*  (See also facing page.)

**2. Hip and Knee Warm-Up**  *(p. 38)*

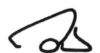

**4. Forward Bends**  *(p. 150)*

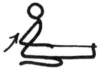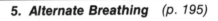

**3. Rock and Roll**  *(p. 94)*

**5. Alternate Breathing**  *(p. 195)*

## THIRTY-MINUTE PROGRAM

**1. Sun Salutation**  *(p. 71)*  (See also facing page.)

**2. Hip and Knee Warm-Ups**  *(p. 38)*

**4. Sit-Balances**  *(p. 66)*

**3. Leg Raises**  *(p. 22)*

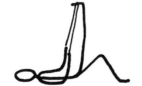

**5. Head Stand**  *(p. 76)*

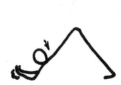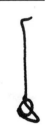

**6. Crossed Leg Rock and Roll** *(p. 96)*

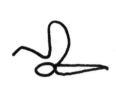

**7. Shoulder Stand** *(p. 106)*

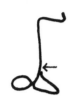  

**8. Cobra** *(p. 114)*

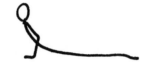

**9. Forward Bends** *(p. 150)*

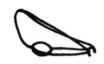  

**10. Alternate Breathing** *(p. 195)*

## MORNING SCHEDULE

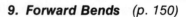 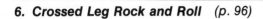 

**1. Sun Salutation** *(p. 71)*

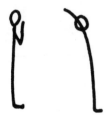 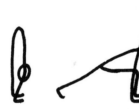  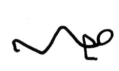

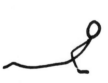 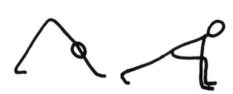 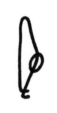 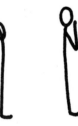

**2. Chest Expander Pose** *(p. 25)*

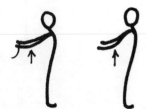

**3. Hip and Knee Warm-Up** *(p. 38)*

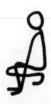

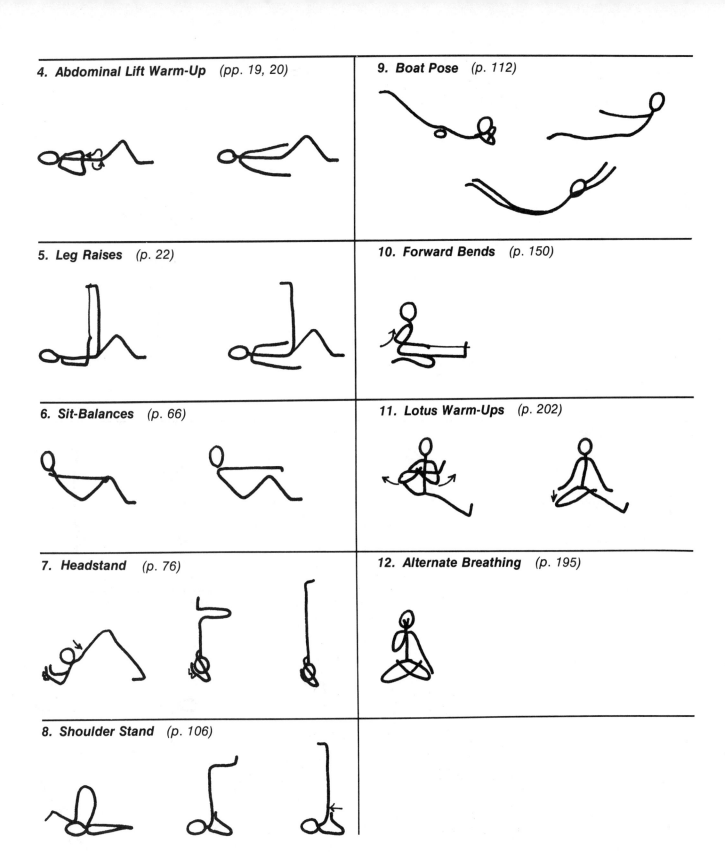

**4. Abdominal Lift Warm-Up**   *(pp. 19, 20)*

**9. Boat Pose**   *(p. 112)*

**5. Leg Raises**   *(p. 22)*

**10. Forward Bends**   *(p. 150)*

**6. Sit-Balances**   *(p. 66)*

**11. Lotus Warm-Ups**   *(p. 202)*

**7. Headstand**   *(p. 76)*

**12. Alternate Breathing**   *(p. 195)*

**8. Shoulder Stand**   *(p. 106)*

213

### 1. Sun Salutation   *(p. 71)*

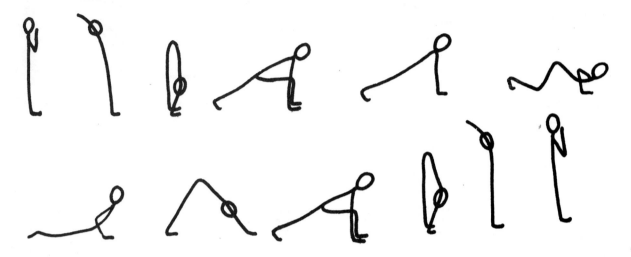

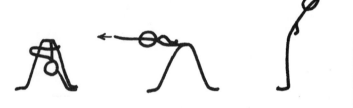

### 2. Pendulum Pose   *(p. 40)*

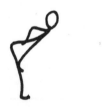  

### 5. Headstand   *(p. 76)*

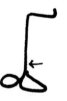 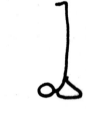

### 3. Split Forward Bends   *(p. 44)*

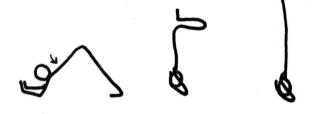

### 6. Shoulder Stand   *(p. 106)*

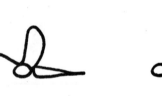

### 4. Intermediate Leg Raises   *(p. 50)*

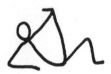 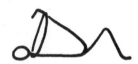

### 7. Cobra Salute   *(p. 117)*

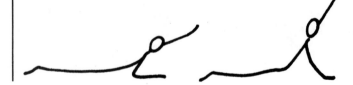

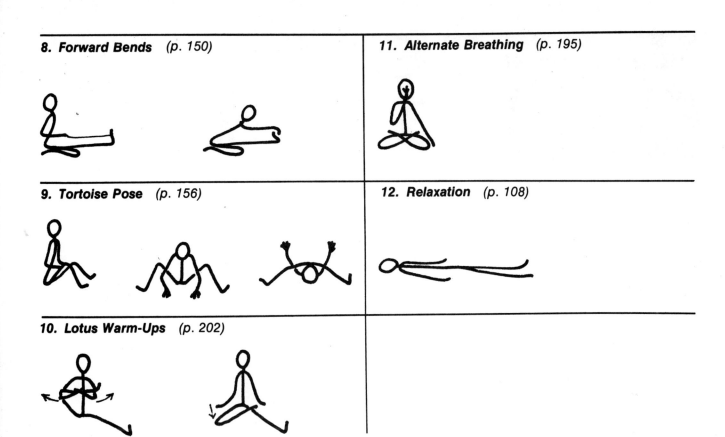

**8. Forward Bends**   *(p. 150)*

**9. Tortoise Pose**   *(p. 156)*

**10. Lotus Warm-Ups**   *(p. 202)*

**11. Alternate Breathing**   *(p. 195)*

**12. Relaxation**   *(p. 108)*

# 25 THERE'S NO EXCUSE

Hatha Yoga can be practiced by every age group, with beneficial results if common sense is used in the approach. If a posture causes discomfort, go back to the beginning and *gently* proceed into it, relaxing within the pose. Go only as far as is comfortable.

Youngsters and teenagers derive benefits from Hatha Yoga, attaining coordination and motor skills in a non-competitive setting. For the child who can not make the team, individual achievement can help to bring poise and a good self-image. For all children, the breathing and flexibility are good warm-ups for competitive sports.

Expectant mothers can have better circulation and fewer leg and back complaints, in addition to a body that is better prepared for delivery if they practice Hatha Yoga during pregnancy.

Working adults can adapt Hatha Yoga to their schedules and attire and very possibly forego the "coffee break" for a few relaxing breaths and stretches.

All the foregoing reasons for practicing Hatha Yoga apply doubly to senior citizens. Relaxation and good breathing can help make the later years more pleasant, for as flexibility and circulation improves, the body becomes rejuvenated and the mind more alert. Always check with the doctor before embarking on an exercise program, and then proceed gently. Age itself is not a limiting factor. I have had students 80 years old. Remember that "You are as young as your spine is supple."

So there's *no excuse*. Try Hatha Yoga.

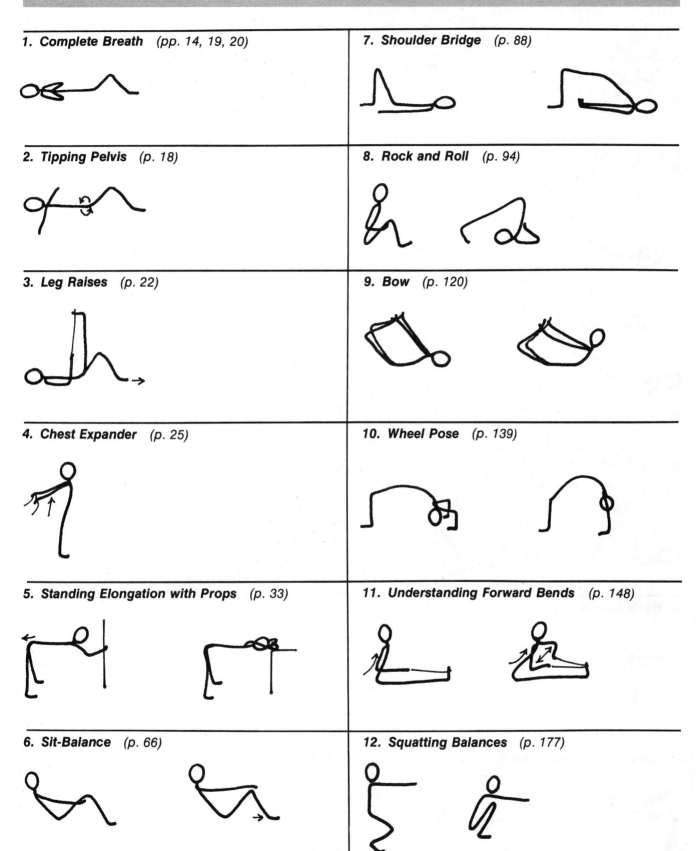

**1. Complete Breath**  (pp. 14, 19, 20)

**2. Tipping Pelvis**  (p. 18)

**3. Leg Raises**  (p. 22)

**4. Chest Expander**  (p. 25)

**5. Standing Elongation with Props**  (p. 33)

**6. Sit-Balance**  (p. 66)

**7. Shoulder Bridge**  (p. 88)

**8. Rock and Roll**  (p. 94)

**9. Bow**  (p. 120)

**10. Wheel Pose**  (p. 139)

**11. Understanding Forward Bends**  (p. 148)

**12. Squatting Balances**  (p. 177)

**13. Lotus Warm-Up** *(p. 202)*

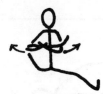

**14. Alternate Breathing** *(p. 195)*

## YOGA FOR TEENAGERS

**1. Complete Breath** *(pp. 14, 19)*

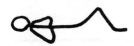

**6. Sit-Downs and Ups** *(p. 68)*

**2. Tummy-In Technique** *(p. 20)*

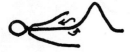

**7. Head Stand Warm-Ups** *(p. 74)*

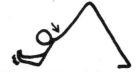

**3. Leg Raises** *(p. 22)*

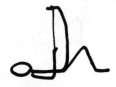
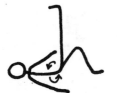

**8. Neck Tilt and Stretch** *(pp. 86, 87)*

**4. Blade Squeeze** *(p. 26)*

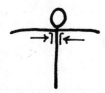

**9. Plough Pose** *(p. 98)*

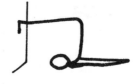
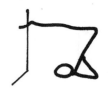

**5. Elongating Legs and Back** *(p. 36)*

**10. Shoulder Stand** *(p. 106)*

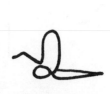
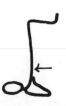
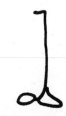

218

**11. Locust** *(p. 118)*

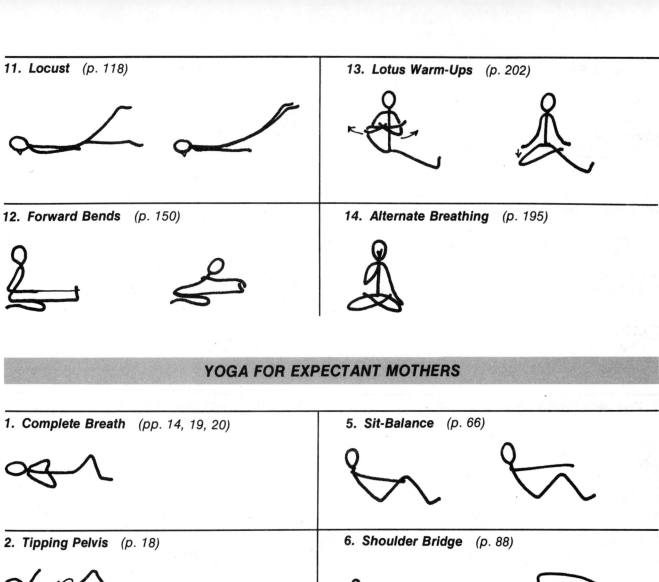

**12. Forward Bends** *(p. 150)*

**13. Lotus Warm-Ups** *(p. 202)*

**14. Alternate Breathing** *(p. 195)*

## YOGA FOR EXPECTANT MOTHERS

**1. Complete Breath** *(pp. 14, 19, 20)*

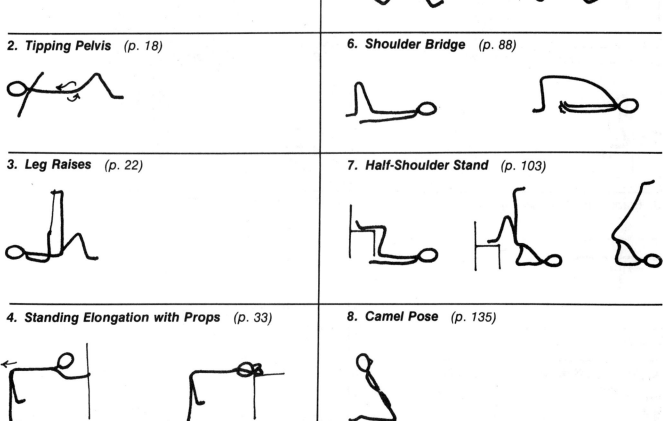

**2. Tipping Pelvis** *(p. 18)*

**3. Leg Raises** *(p. 22)*

**4. Standing Elongation with Props** *(p. 33)*

**5. Sit-Balance** *(p. 66)*

**6. Shoulder Bridge** *(p. 88)*

**7. Half-Shoulder Stand** *(p. 103)*

**8. Camel Pose** *(p. 135)*

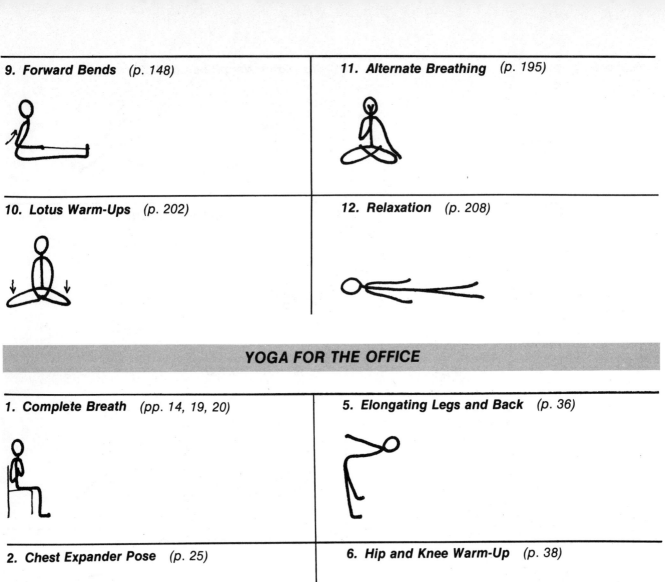

**9. Forward Bends** *(p. 148)*

**11. Alternate Breathing** *(p. 195)*

**10. Lotus Warm-Ups** *(p. 202)*

**12. Relaxation** *(p. 208)*

## YOGA FOR THE OFFICE

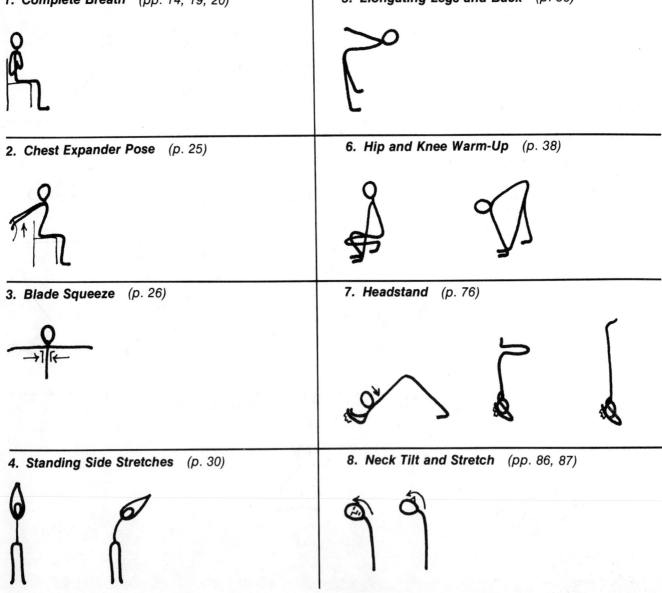

**1. Complete Breath** *(pp. 14, 19, 20)*

**5. Elongating Legs and Back** *(p. 36)*

**2. Chest Expander Pose** *(p. 25)*

**6. Hip and Knee Warm-Up** *(p. 38)*

**3. Blade Squeeze** *(p. 26)*

**7. Headstand** *(p. 76)*

**4. Standing Side Stretches** *(p. 30)*

**8. Neck Tilt and Stretch** *(pp. 86, 87)*

**9. Forward Bends**  *(p. 250)*

**10. Push-Ups**  *(pp. 183 or 184)*

**11. Alternate Breathing**  *(p. 195)*

**12. Relaxation in Chair**  *(p. 208)*

## YOGA FOR SENIOR CITIZENS

**1. Complete Breath**  *(p. 14)*

**2. Chest Expander**  *(p. 25)*

**3. Blade Squeeze**  *(p. 26)*

**4. Abdominal Lift Warm-Up**  *(p. 19)*

**5. Tummy-In Technique**  *(p. 20)*

**6. Leg Raises**  *(p. 22)*

**7. Hip and Knee Warm-Ups**  *(p. 38)*

**8. Neck Tilt and Stretch**  *(pp. 86, 87)*

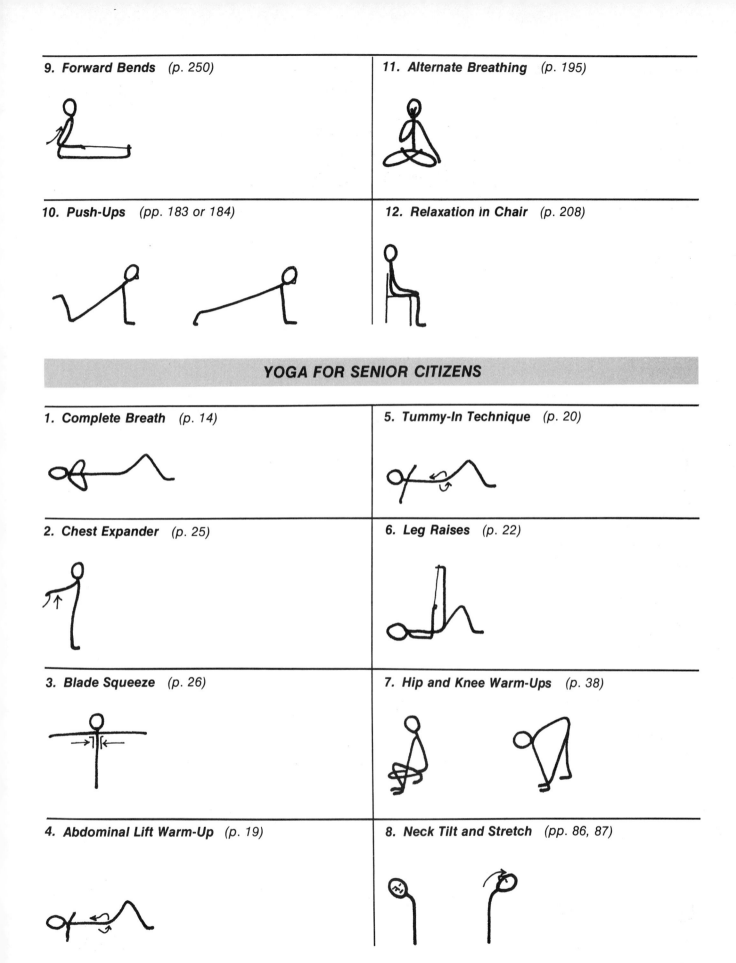

**9. Half-Shoulder Stand with Chair**   *(p. 104)*

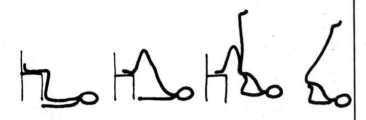

**11. Understanding Forward Bends**   *(p. 148)*

**10. Boat Pose**   *(p. 112)*

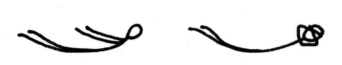

**12. Alternate Breathing**   *(p. 195)*

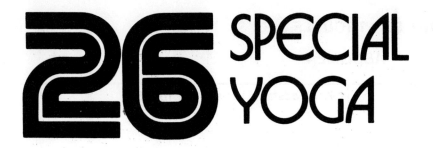

# 26 SPECIAL YOGA

These Hatha Yoga exercises are suggestions only and should never be substituted for medical treatment. Be sure to consult your physician if you have any questions about the effect of following these exercise programs. Experience has shown that many doctors recommend this type of exercise for their patients.

Hatha Yoga is excellent for the sportsperson. Yoga breathing is an asset to any sports program. The vigorous repetitious movements involved in sports tend to overdevelop one side or area of the body, thus inviting a serious disproportion. The flexibility gained from doing the postures makes for a good limbering warm-up and helps to offset any strain incurred by sports.

Ahead are some of the Trouble Spots on which some people need extra help in order to participate in a sport, or because one area of the body needs help. Remember that Hatha Yoga increases blood circulation to the surrounding area of the part which is being exercised, so if there is not a specific posture for a Trouble Spot, do one that works on the next closest area. Specific sports which are helped by Hatha Yoga are gymnastics, hockey, soccer, football, baseball, golf, skiing and tennis. These are a mere handful. Whatever the sport, Hatha Yoga can help in the warm-up, the play, and the post-game slow down.

## ABDOMEN

**1. Abdominal Lift Warm-Up**  *(pp. 19, 20)*

**7. Headstand Variations**  *(p. 78)*

**2. Tent Pose**  *(p. 42)*

**8. Plough Pose**  *(p. 98)*

**3. Scissor Swing**  *(p. 56)*

**9. Shoulder Stand Variations**  *(p. 108)*

**4. Gut Balance**  *(p. 60)*

**10. Hydrant Pose**  *(p. 131)*

**5. Sit-Balance**  *(p. 66)*

**11. Angle Balances**  *(p. 174)*

**6. Sit-Downs and-Ups**  *(pp. 68, 69)*

**12. Abdominal Lift**  *(p. 198)*

ANKLES AND FEET

**1. Raise Toes and Kneecaps**  *(pp. 7, 8)*

**2. Plough Pose**  *(p. 98)*

**3. Closed Bow**  *(p. 122)*

**4. Nut Cracker**  *(p. 128)*

**5. Camel Pose**  *(p. 135)*

**6. Kneeling Pose**  *(p. 136)*

**7. Forward Bends**  *(p. 150)*

**8. Squatting Balances**  *(p. 177)*

**9. Flamingo Pose**  *(p. 179)*

**10. Lotus Warm-Ups**  *(p. 202)*

ARMS AND SHOULDERS

**1. Chest Expander Pose**  *(p. 25)*

**2. Blade Pose**  *(p. 26)*

225

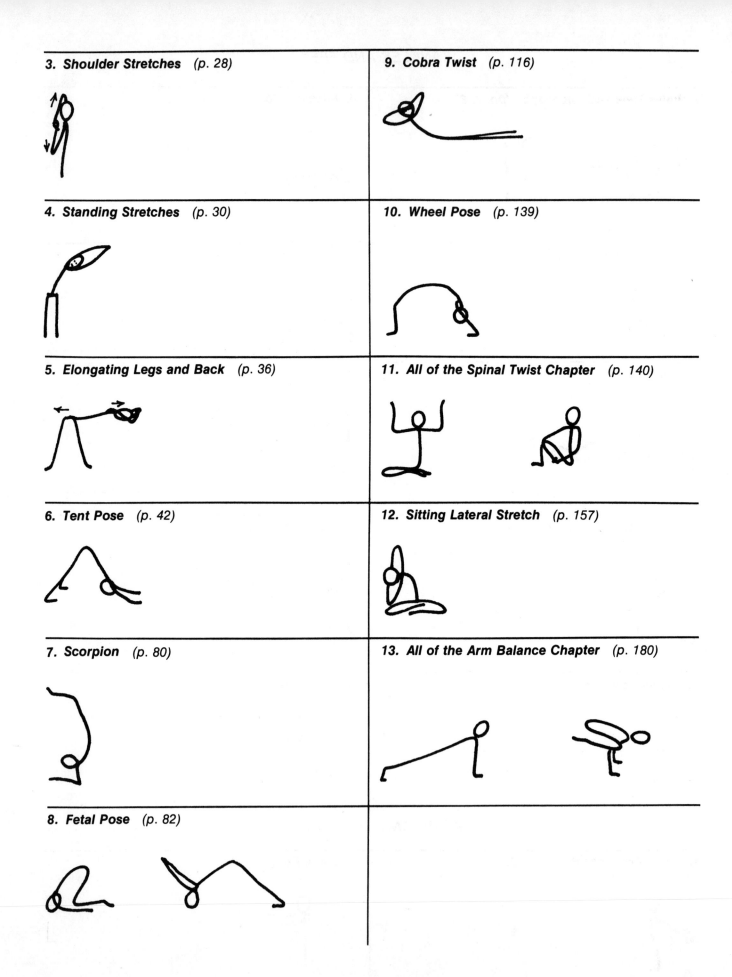

**3. Shoulder Stretches** *(p. 28)*

**4. Standing Stretches** *(p. 30)*

**5. Elongating Legs and Back** *(p. 36)*

**6. Tent Pose** *(p. 42)*

**7. Scorpion** *(p. 80)*

**8. Fetal Pose** *(p. 82)*

**9. Cobra Twist** *(p. 116)*

**10. Wheel Pose** *(p. 139)*

**11. All of the Spinal Twist Chapter** *(p. 140)*

**12. Sitting Lateral Stretch** *(p. 157)*

**13. All of the Arm Balance Chapter** *(p. 180)*

**1. Read "Getting to Know Your Body"**  *(p. 6)*

**2. All of the Abdomen & Pelvis Chapter**  *(p. 16)*

**3. Standing Elongation with Props**  *(p. 33)*

**8. Shoulder Stand**  *(p. 106)*

**4. Hip and Knee Warm-Ups**  *(p. 38)*

**9. Boat Pose**  *(p. 112)*

**5. Sit-Downs and-Ups**  *(p. 69)*

**10. All of the Spinal Twist Chapter**  *(p. 140)*

**6. Shoulder Bridge**  *(p. 88)*

**11. All of the Sitting Forward Bends Chapter**
    *(p. 146)*

**7. Plough Pose**  *(p. 98)*

**12. All of the Standing Balances Chapter**  *(p. 158)*

**1. Hip and Knee Warm-Ups** *(p. 38)*

**7. Ostrich** *(p. 101)*

**2. Elongating Legs & Back** *(p. 36)*

**8. Shoulder Stand Variations** *(p. 108)*

**3. Tent Pose** *(p. 42)*

**9. Locust Pose** *(p. 118)*

**4. Intermediate Leg Raises** *(p. 50)*

**10. Hydrant Pose** *(p. 131)*

**5. Headstand Variations** *(p. 78)*

**11. Pigeon Pose** *(p. 129)*

**6. Bridge Extension** *(p. 92)*

**12. Vise Pose** *(p. 137)*

**13. Forward Bends**  *(p. 150)*

**14. Dancer #2 Position**  *(p. 160)*

**15. Lotus Warm-Up**  *(p. 202)*

**16. Lotus Posture**  *(p. 204)*

## NECK AND CHIN

**1. Chest Expander**  *(p. 25)*

**2. Headstand**  *(p. 76)*

**3. Fetal Pose**  *(p. 82)*

**4. Neck Tilt**  *(p. 86)*

**5. Neck Stretch**  *(p. 87)*

**6. Head Bridge**  *(p. 90)*

**7. Lunging Forward Bends**  *(p. 126)*

**8. Frog Pose**  *(p. 133)*

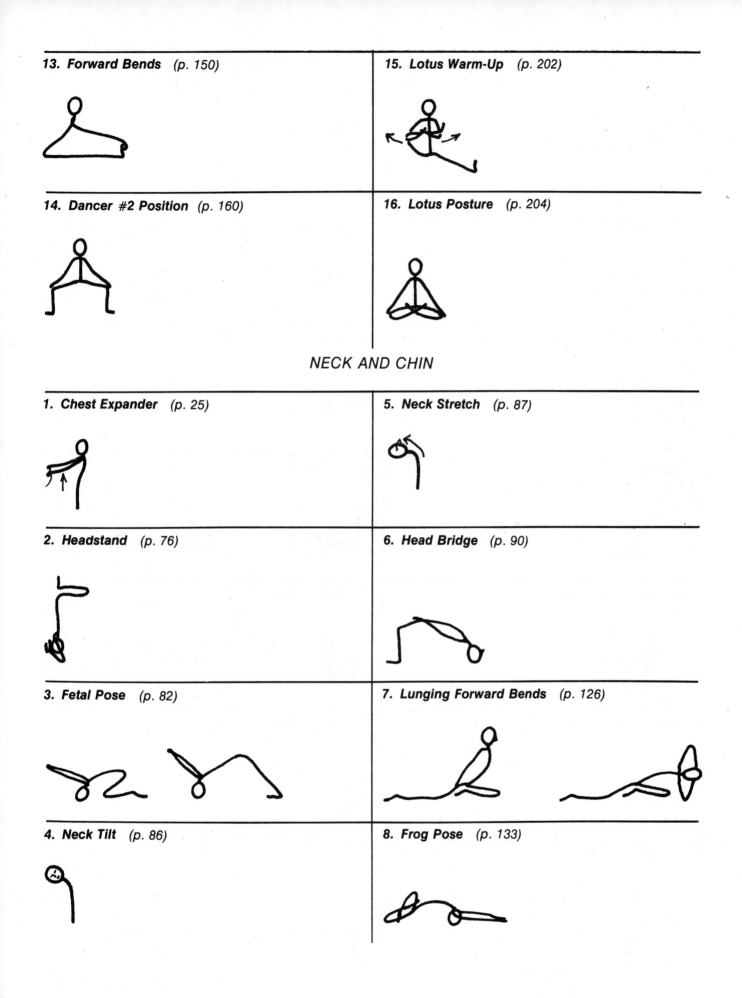

**9. Fish** *(p. 134)*

**10. All of the Spinal Twist chapter** *(p. 140)*

## WAIST

**1. Abdominal Lift Warm-Up** *(pp. 19, 20)*

**7. Advanced Rock and Roll** *(p. 100)*

**2. Elongating Legs and Back** *(p. 36)*

**8. Hydrant Pose** *(p. 131)*

**3. Tent Pose** *(p. 42)*

**9. Kneeling Bridge Pose** *(p. 138)*

**4. Pendulum Leg Swing** *(p. 58)*

**10. Spinal Twist** *(p. 145)*

**5. Sit Balances** *(p. 66)*

**11. Sitting Lateral Stretch** *(p. 157)*

**6. Pin Wheel** *(p. 91)*

**12. Abdominal Lift** *(p. 198)*

**1. Complete Breath**   *(p. 14)*

**2. Abdominal Lift Warm-Ups**   *(pp. 19, 20)*

**3. Leg Raises**   *(p. 22)*

**4. Chest Expander Pose**   *(p. 25)*

**5. Standing Elongation with Props**   *(p. 33)*

**6. Neck Tilt and Stretch**   *(pp. 86, 87)*

**7. Half-Shoulder Stand**   *(p. 103)*

**8. Rock and Roll**   *(p. 94)*

**9. Frog Pose**   *(p. 133)*

**10. Twist Warm-Up with Wall**   *(p. 141)*

**11. Fetal Pose**   *(p. 82)*

**12. Alternate Breathing and Relaxation**   *(pp. 195, 208)*

## ARTHRITIS

**1. Chest Expander Pose**  (p. 25)

**7. Rock and Roll**  (p. 94)

**2. Blade Squeeze Pose**  (p. 26)

**8. Closed Bow**  (p. 122)

**3. Shoulder Stretches**  (p. 28)

**9. Frog Pose**  (p. 133)

**4. Hip and Knee Warm-Up**  (p. 38)

**10. Twist Warm-Up with Wall**  (p. 140)

**5. Fetal Pose**  (p. 82)

**11. Squatting Balance**  (p. 177)

**6. Shoulder Bridge**  (p. 88)

**12. Lotus Warm-Ups**  (p. 202)

**1. Abdominal Lift Warm-Up** *(pp. 19, 20)*

**7. Plough Pose** *(p. 98)*

**2. Leg Raises** *(p. 22)*

**8. Boat Pose** *(p. 112)*

**3. Standing Elongation with Props** *(p. 33)*

**9. Fetal Pose** *(p. 82)*

**4. Hip and Knee Warm-Up** *(p. 38)*

**10. Forward Bends** *(p. 148)*

**5. Hip Balance** *(p. 54)*

**11. Abdominal Lift** *(p. 198)*

**6. Sit Balance** *(p. 66)*

**12. Relaxation** *(p. 208)*

**1. Abdominal Lift Warm-Ups** *(pp. 19, 20)*

**2. Hip and Knee Warm-Up** *(p. 38)*

**3. Sun Salutation** *(p. 71)*

**4. Crossed Leg Rock and Roll** *(p. 96)*

**6. Spinal Twist** *(p. 145)*

**5. Bow Pose** *(p. 120)*

**7. Forward Bends** *(p. 150)*

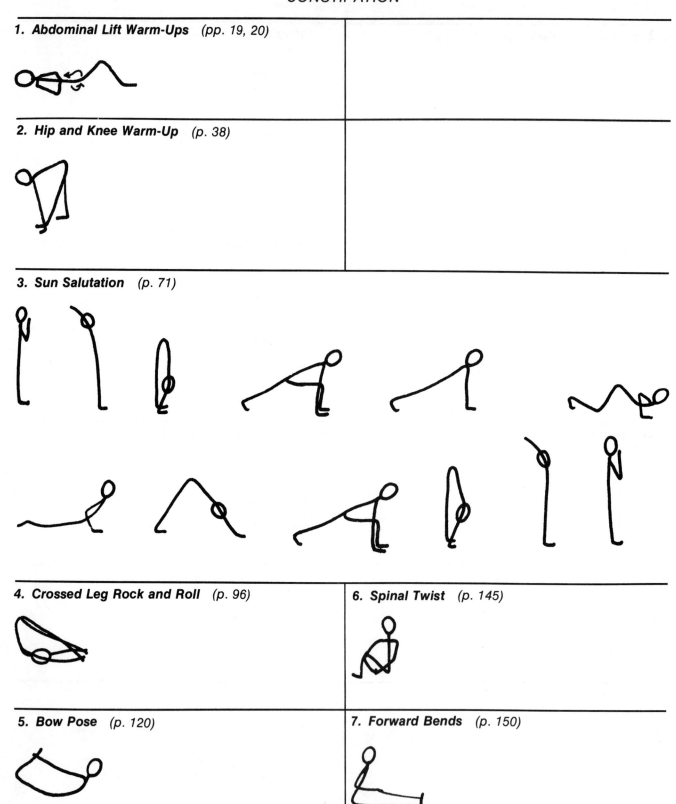

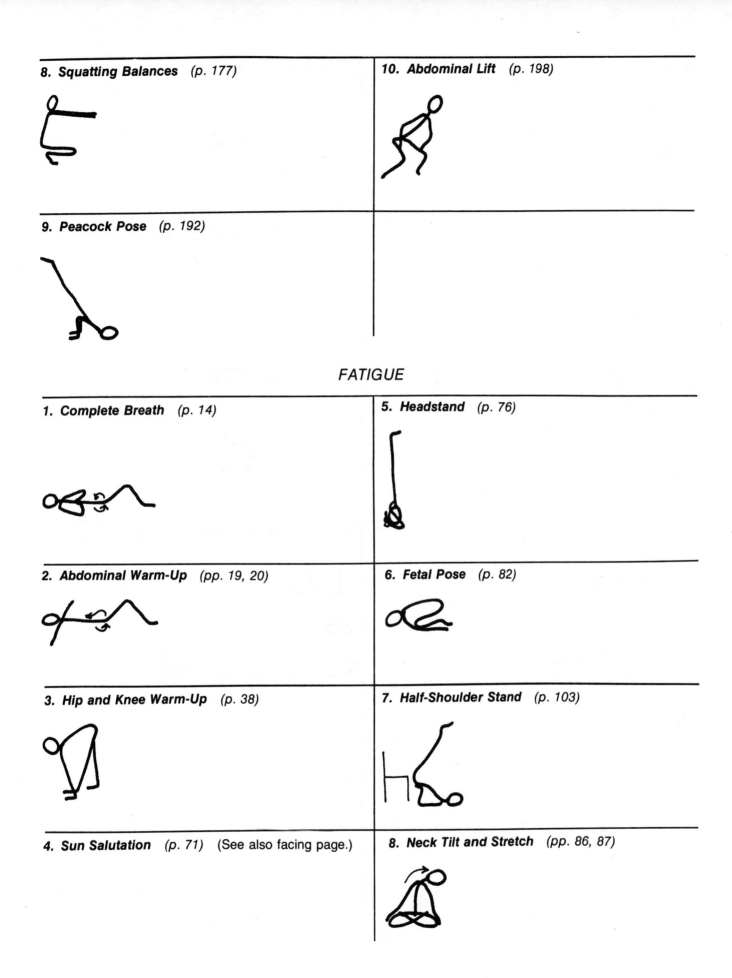

**8. Squatting Balances** *(p. 177)*

**10. Abdominal Lift** *(p. 198)*

**9. Peacock Pose** *(p. 192)*

## FATIGUE

**1. Complete Breath** *(p. 14)*

**5. Headstand** *(p. 76)*

**2. Abdominal Warm-Up** *(pp. 19, 20)*

**6. Fetal Pose** *(p. 82)*

**3. Hip and Knee Warm-Up** *(p. 38)*

**7. Half-Shoulder Stand** *(p. 103)*

**4. Sun Salutation** *(p. 71)* (See also facing page.)

**8. Neck Tilt and Stretch** *(pp. 86, 87)*

**9. All of the Breathing Technique chapter** *(p. 193)*

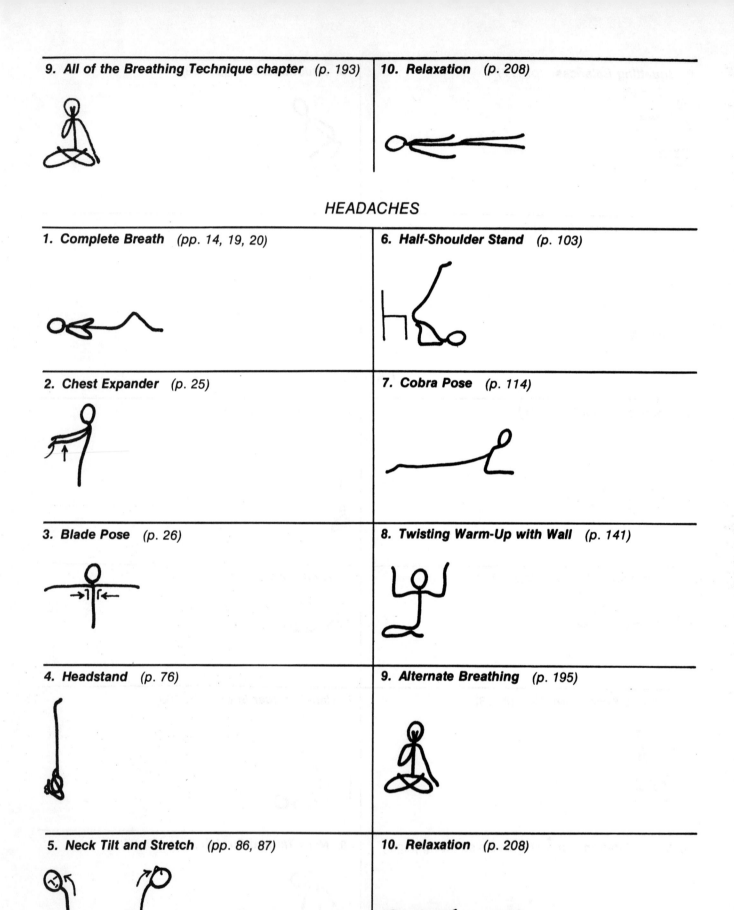

**10. Relaxation** *(p. 208)*

## HEADACHES

**1. Complete Breath** *(pp. 14, 19, 20)*

**6. Half-Shoulder Stand** *(p. 103)*

**2. Chest Expander** *(p. 25)*

**7. Cobra Pose** *(p. 114)*

**3. Blade Pose** *(p. 26)*

**8. Twisting Warm-Up with Wall** *(p. 141)*

**4. Headstand** *(p. 76)*

**9. Alternate Breathing** *(p. 195)*

**5. Neck Tilt and Stretch** *(pp. 86, 87)*

**10. Relaxation** *(p. 208)*

**1. Complete Breath**   *(pp. 14, 19, 20)*

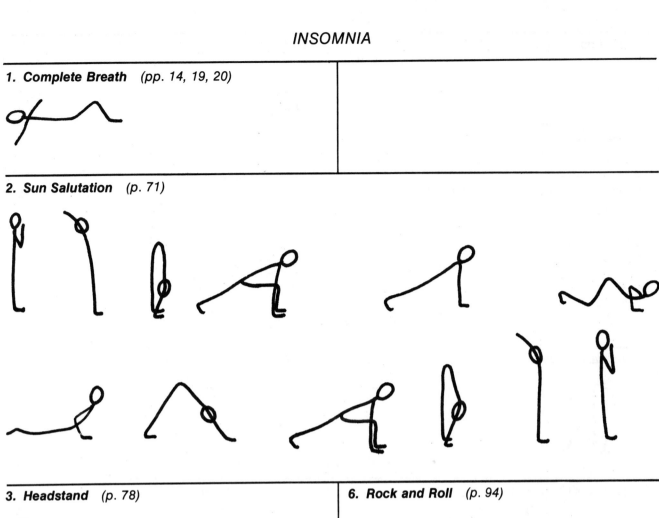

**2. Sun Salutation**   *(p. 71)*

**3. Headstand**   *(p. 78)*

**6. Rock and Roll**   *(p. 94)*

**4. Fetal Pose**   *(p. 82)*

**7. Shoulder Stand**   *(p. 104)*

**5. Neck Tilt and Stretch**   *(pp. 86, 87)*

**8. Cobra Pose**   *(p. 114)*

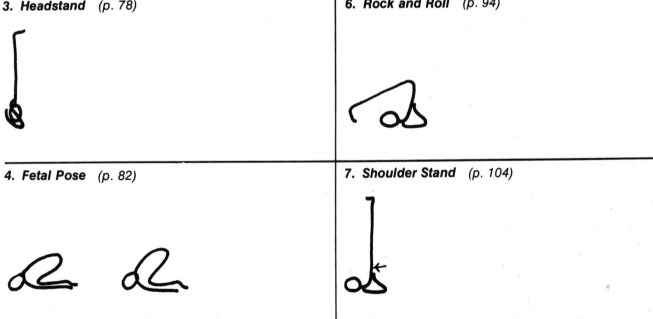

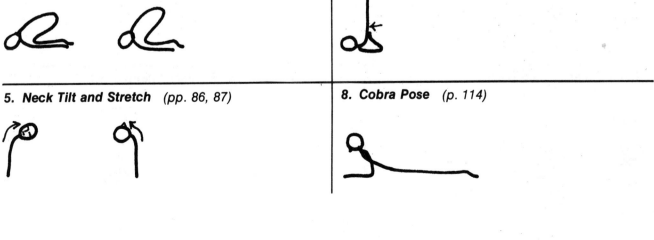

**9. Fish Pose** *(p. 134)*

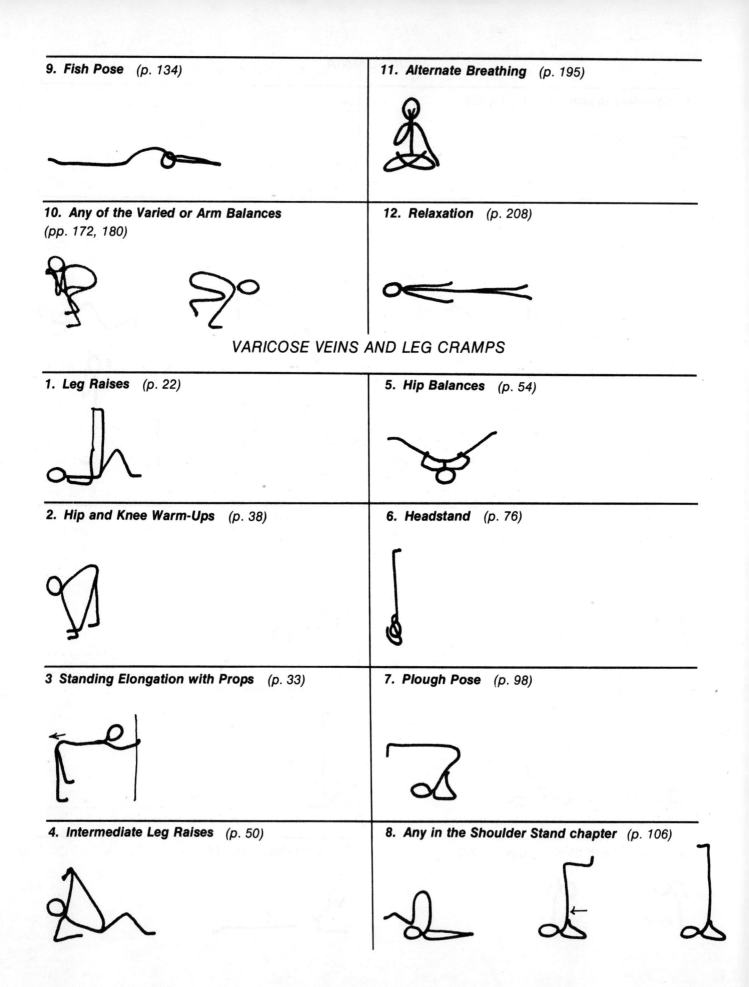

**11. Alternate Breathing** *(p. 195)*

**10. Any of the Varied or Arm Balances** *(pp. 172, 180)*

**12. Relaxation** *(p. 208)*

## VARICOSE VEINS AND LEG CRAMPS

**1. Leg Raises** *(p. 22)*

**5. Hip Balances** *(p. 54)*

**2. Hip and Knee Warm-Ups** *(p. 38)*

**6. Headstand** *(p. 76)*

**3 Standing Elongation with Props** *(p. 33)*

**7. Plough Pose** *(p. 98)*

**4. Intermediate Leg Raises** *(p. 50)*

**8. Any in the Shoulder Stand chapter** *(p. 106)*

**9. Locust** (p. 118)

**11. Squatting Balances** (p. 177)

**10. Forward Bends** (p. 150)

**12. Relaxation** (p. 208)

## WEIGHT CONTROL

**1. Complete Breath** (p. 14)

**5. Tent Pose** (p. 42)

**2. Abdominal Lift Warm-Up** (pp. 19, 20)

**6. Scissor Swing** (p. 56)

**3. Standing Side Stretches** (p. 30)

**7. Gut Balances** . (p. 60)

**4. Hip and Knee Warm-Ups** (p. 38)

**8. Sit-Downs and-Ups** (pp. 68, 69)

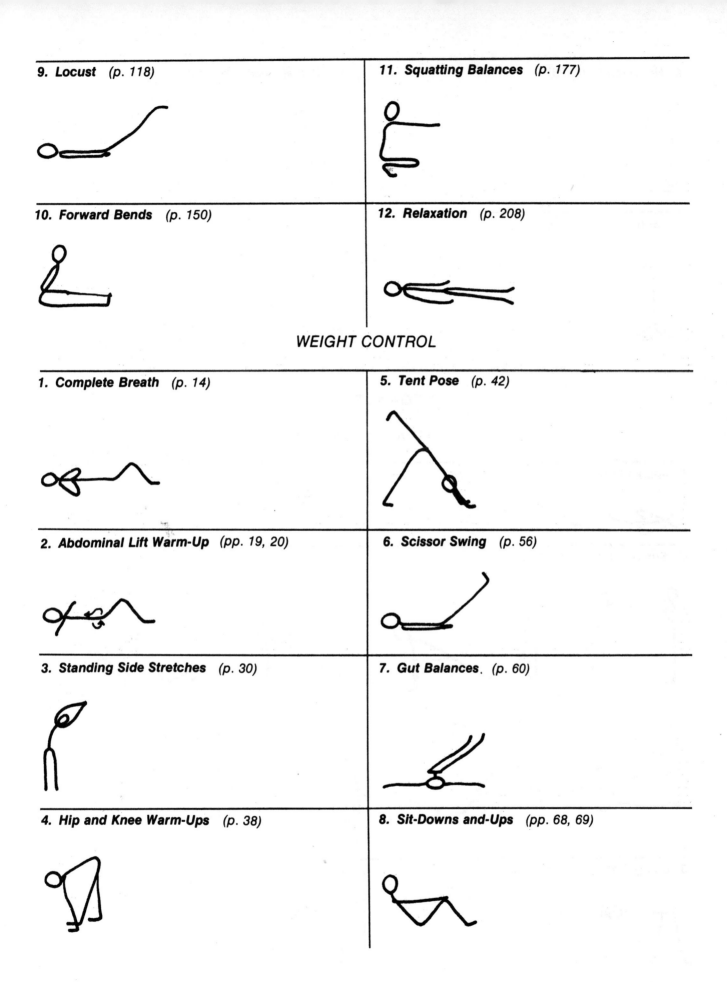

**9. Headstand** *(p. 76)*

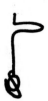

**10. Shoulder Stand** *(p. 106)*

**11. Spinal Twist** *(p. 145)*

**12. Abdominal Lift** *(p. 198)*

## YOGA FOR SPORTS

### GYMNASTIC WARM-UPS

**1. Apply the Complete Breath** *(pp. 14, 19, 20)*

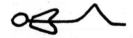

**2. Sun Salutation** *(p. 71)*

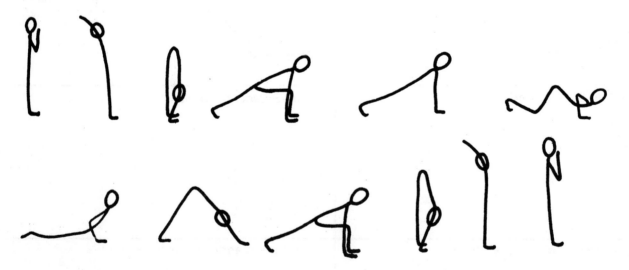

**3. Elongating Legs and Back** *(p. 36)*

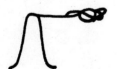

**4. Tent Pose** *(p. 42)*

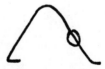

**5. Standing Forward Bends** *(p. 46)*

**6. Advanced Leg Pulls** *(p. 52)*

**7. Rock and Roll with Plough Pose** *(pp. 94, 98)*

**8. Sit-Downs and-Ups** *(pp. 68, 69)*

**9. Scorpion** *(p. 80)*

**10. Lunges** *(p. 124)*

**11. Cobra Twist** *(p. 116)*

**12. Wheel Pose** *(p. 139)*

**13. Advanced Forward Bends** *(p. 154)*

**14. Tortoise Pose** *(p. 156)*

**15. All in the Standing Balances chapter** *(p. 158)*

**16. Push-Ups** *(p. 194)*

241

**17. Side Inclined Plane** *(p. 188)*

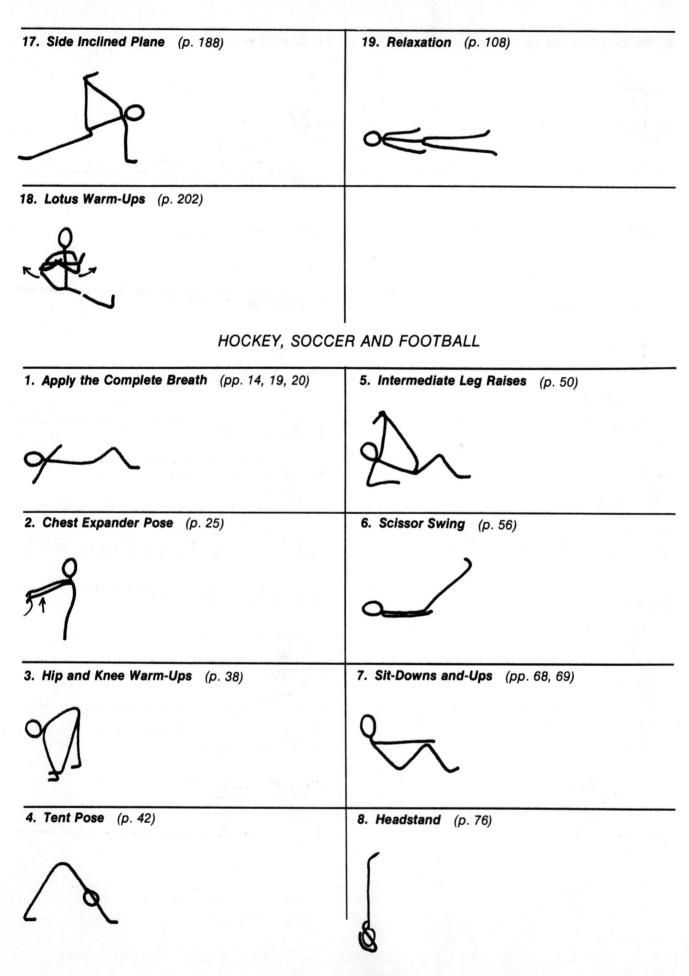

**18. Lotus Warm-Ups** *(p. 202)*

**19. Relaxation** *(p. 108)*

## HOCKEY, SOCCER AND FOOTBALL

**1. Apply the Complete Breath** *(pp. 14, 19, 20)*

**2. Chest Expander Pose** *(p. 25)*

**3. Hip and Knee Warm-Ups** *(p. 38)*

**4. Tent Pose** *(p. 42)*

**5. Intermediate Leg Raises** *(p. 50)*

**6. Scissor Swing** *(p. 56)*

**7. Sit-Downs and-Ups** *(pp. 68, 69)*

**8. Headstand** *(p. 76)*

**9. Neck Tilt and Stretch**  (pp. 86, 87)

**16. Forward Bends**  (p. 150)

**10. Advanced Rock and Roll**  (p. 100)

**17. Squatting Balances**  (p. 177)

**11. Shoulder Stand**  (p. 106)

**18. Push-Ups**  (p. 184)

**12. Cobra Twist**  (p. 116)

**19. Incline Plane**  (p. 196)

**13. Camel Pose**  (p. 135)

**20. Lotus Warm-Ups**  (p. 202)

**14. Vise Press**  (p. 137)

**21. Relaxation**  (p. 208)

**15. Easy Twist**  (p. 142)

**1. Apply the Complete Breath** (pp. 14, 20)
(Inhale on the swing back; exhale upon contact and follow through.)

**2. Chest Expander Pose** (p. 25)

**3. Blade Squeeze** (p. 26)

**4. Standing Side Stretch** (p. 30)

**5. Hip and Knee Warm-Ups** (p. 38)

**6. Pendulum Pose** (p. 40)

**7. Tent Pose** (p. 42)

**8. Intermediate Leg Raises** (p. 50)

**9. Hip Balance** (p. 54)

**10. Sit-Downs and-Ups** (pp. 68, 69)

**11. Neck Tilt and Stretch** (pp. 86, 87)

**12. Rock and Roll** (p. 94)

**13. Boat Pose** *(p. 112)*

**14. Lunge Pose** *(p. 124)*

**15. Fish Pose** *(p. 133)*

**16. Forward Bends** *(p. 150)*

**17. Squatting Balance** *(p. 177)*

**18. Incline Plane** *(p. 186)*

**19. Push-Ups** *(p. 185)*

**20. Lotus Warm-Ups** *(p. 202)*

**21. Relaxation** *(p. 208)*

GOLF

**1. Apply the Complete Breath** *(pp. 14, 20)*
*(Inhale on the up stroke and exhale on the down stroke.)*

**2. Chest Expander Pose** *(p. 25)*

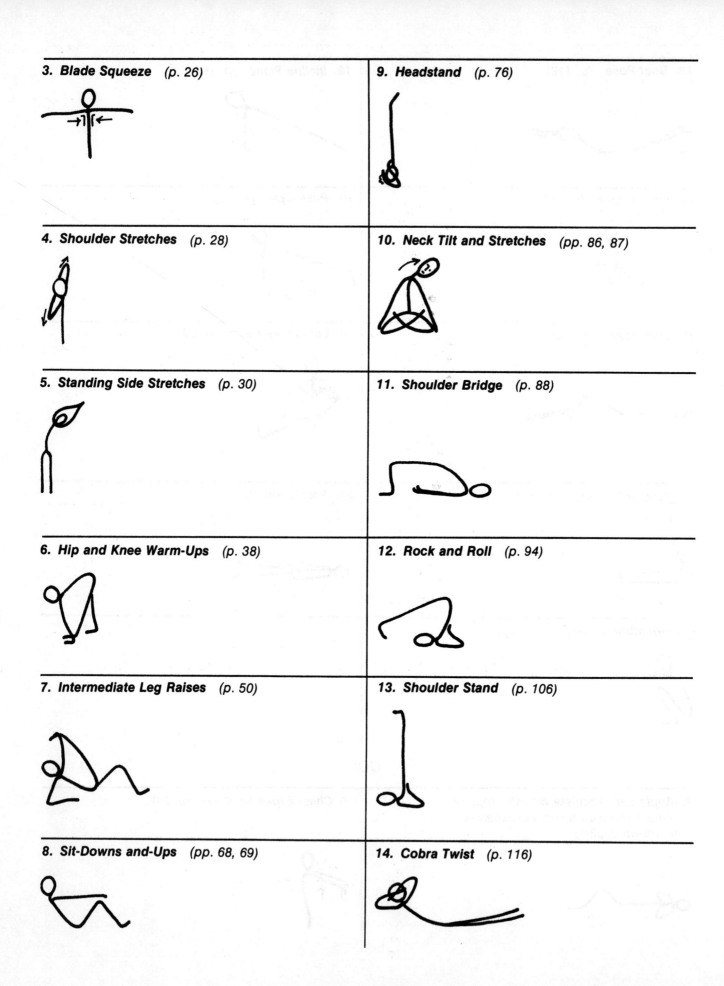

**3. Blade Squeeze** *(p. 26)*

**4. Shoulder Stretches** *(p. 28)*

**5. Standing Side Stretches** *(p. 30)*

**6. Hip and Knee Warm-Ups** *(p. 38)*

**7. Intermediate Leg Raises** *(p. 50)*

**8. Sit-Downs and-Ups** *(pp. 68, 69)*

**9. Headstand** *(p. 76)*

**10. Neck Tilt and Stretches** *(pp. 86, 87)*

**11. Shoulder Bridge** *(p. 88)*

**12. Rock and Roll** *(p. 94)*

**13. Shoulder Stand** *(p. 106)*

**14. Cobra Twist** *(p. 116)*

**15. Cobra Salute**  (p. 117)

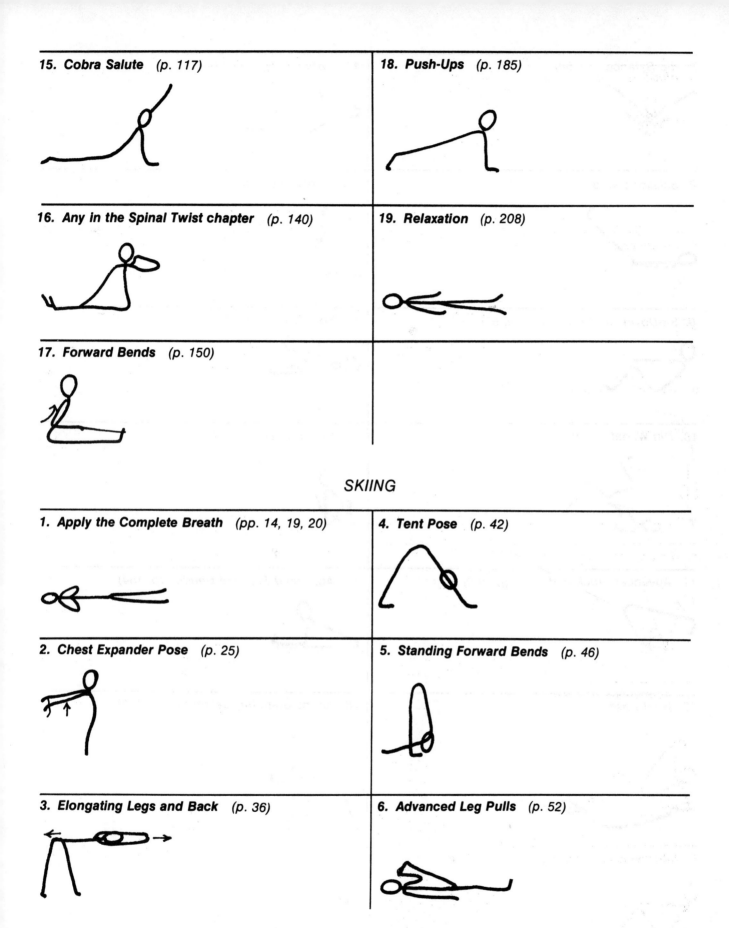

**18. Push-Ups**  (p. 185)

**16. Any in the Spinal Twist chapter**  (p. 140)

**19. Relaxation**  (p. 208)

**17. Forward Bends**  (p. 150)

## SKIING

**1. Apply the Complete Breath**  (pp. 14, 19, 20)

**4. Tent Pose**  (p. 42)

**2. Chest Expander Pose**  (p. 25)

**5. Standing Forward Bends**  (p. 46)

**3. Elongating Legs and Back**  (p. 36)

**6. Advanced Leg Pulls**  (p. 52)

**7. Hip Balance**   *(p. 54)*

**8. Scissor Swing**   *(p. 56)*

**9. Sit-Downs and-Ups**   *(pp. 68, 69)*

**10. Pin Wheel**   *(p. 91)*

**11. Advanced Rock and Roll**   *(p. 100)*

**12. Boat Pose**   *(p. 112)*

**13. Cobra Twist**   *(p. 116)*

**14. Camel Pose**   *(p. 135)*

**15. Vise Press**   *(p. 137)*

**16. Spinal Twist**   *(p. 145)*

**17. Advanced Forward Bends**   *(p. 154)*

**18. All the Standing Balances**   *(p. 158)*

**19. Squatting Balance**  *(p. 177)*

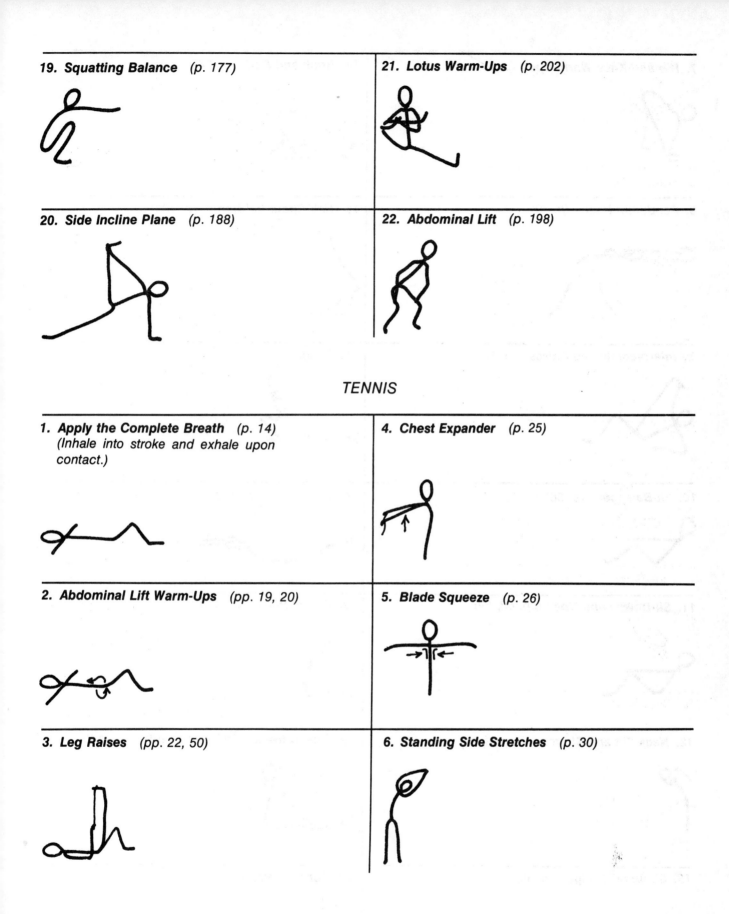

**20. Side Incline Plane**  *(p. 188)*

**21. Lotus Warm-Ups**  *(p. 202)*

**22. Abdominal Lift**  *(p. 198)*

## TENNIS

**1. Apply the Complete Breath**  *(p. 14)*
*(Inhale into stroke and exhale upon contact.)*

**2. Abdominal Lift Warm-Ups**  *(pp. 19, 20)*

**3. Leg Raises**  *(pp. 22, 50)*

**4. Chest Expander**  *(p. 25)*

**5. Blade Squeeze**  *(p. 26)*

**6. Standing Side Stretches**  *(p. 30)*

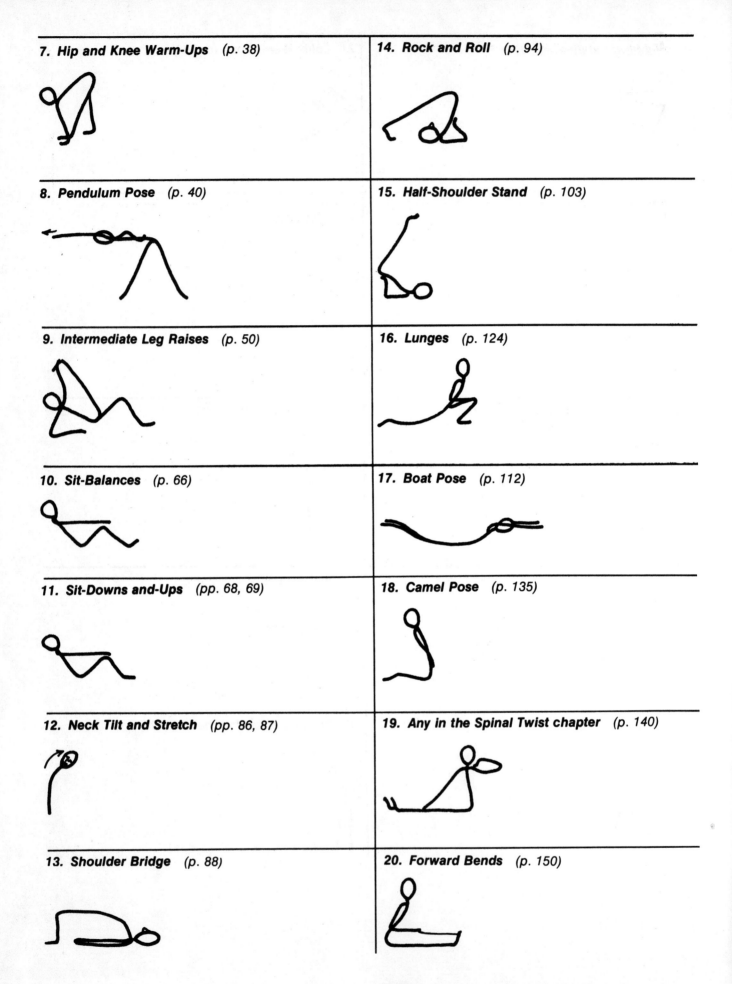

7. **Hip and Knee Warm-Ups**   (p. 38)

8. **Pendulum Pose**   (p. 40)

9. **Intermediate Leg Raises**   (p. 50)

10. **Sit-Balances**   (p. 66)

11. **Sit-Downs and-Ups**   (pp. 68, 69)

12. **Neck Tilt and Stretch**   (pp. 86, 87)

13. **Shoulder Bridge**   (p. 88)

14. **Rock and Roll**   (p. 94)

15. **Half-Shoulder Stand**   (p. 103)

16. **Lunges**   (p. 124)

17. **Boat Pose**   (p. 112)

18. **Camel Pose**   (p. 135)

19. **Any in the Spinal Twist chapter**   (p. 140)

20. **Forward Bends**   (p. 150)

**21. Any of the Standing Balances**  *(p. 158)*

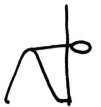

**22. Incline Plane**  *(p. 186)*

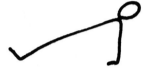

**23. Push-Ups**  *(p. 185)*

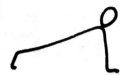

**24. Relaxation**  *(p. 208)*

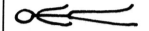

# SELECTED
# REFERENCES

Evans, William F. *Anatomy and Physiology,* Englewood Cliffs, N.J.: Prentice-Hall, Inc., 1976.

Feldenkrais, Moshe. *Awareness Through Movement*. New York: Harper and Row, 1972.

Friedmann, Lawrence W., and Lawrence Galton. *Freedom from Back-Aches*. New York: Simon and Schuster, 1973.

Iyengar, B. K. S. *Light On Yoga*. New York: Schocken Books, 1975.

Kelley, David L. *Kinesiology: Fundamentals of Motion Description*. Englewood Cliffs, N.J.: Prentice-Hall, Inc., 1971.

Lagerwerff, Ellen B., and Karen A. Perlroth. *Mensendieck Your Posture and Your Pains*. New York: Anchor Press/Doubleday, 1973.

Luby, Sue. *Yoga Is For You*. Englewood Cliffs, N.J.: Prentice-Hall, Inc., 1974.

Luby, Sue. *"Hatha Yoga For Total Health",* a double record album, 1976. Box 254, Andover, Mass., 01810. Also available in cassette.

Michele, Arthur A. *Orthotherapy*. New York: M. Evans & Co., Inc., 1971.

Oki, Masahiro. *Practical Yoga: A Pictorial Approach*. Tokyo: Japan Publications, Inc., 1970.

Rasch, Philip J., and Roger K. Burke. *Kinesiology and Applied Anatomy: The Science of Human Movement*. Philadelphia: Lea & Febiger, 1974.

Roberts, Elizabeth H. *On Your Feet*. Emmaus, Pa.: Rodale Press, 1975.

Yesudian, Selvarajan, and Elisabeth Haich. *Yoga and Health*. New York: Harper & Row, 1953.

# INDEX